Natural Healing
for
Dogs

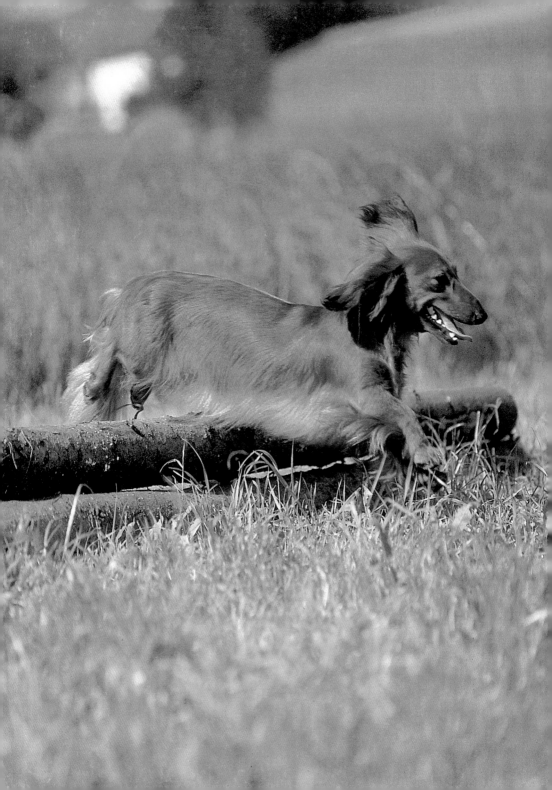

Natural Healing
for
Dogs

Susanne Bönisch

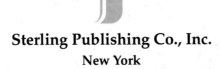

Sterling Publishing Co., Inc.
New York

Contents

Photos: Monika Wegler, Munich

Illustrations: Bettina Buresch, Munich

Translation by Elisabeth Reinersmann

T 52h09S90 280b E

Library of Congress Cataloging-in-Publication Data

Bönisch, Susanne.
  [Hunde natürlich heilen. English]
  Natural healing for dogs / Susanne Bönisch.
    p. cm.
  Includes index.
  ISBN 0-8069-8120-2
  1. Veterinary alternative medicine.   2. Dogs—Diseases—
Alternative treatment.   I. Title.
SF745.5.B6513 1996
636.7'08953—dc20   96-19222
                                                CIP

10 9 8 7 6 5 4 3 2 1

Published 1996 by Sterling Publishing Company, Inc.
387 Park Avenue South, New York, N.Y. 10016
Originally published by Mosaic Verlag GmbH, Munich
under the title *Hunde Natürlich Heilen*
© 1994 by Mosaic Verlag
English translation © 1996 by Sterling Publishing Co., Inc.
Distributed in Canada by Sterling Publishing
℅ Canadian Manda Group, One Atlantic Avenue, Suite 105
Toronto, Ontario, Canada M6K 3E7
Distributed in Great Britain and Europe by Cassell PLC
Wellington House, 125 Strand, London WC2R 0BB, England
Distributed in Australia by Capricorn Link (Australia) Pty Ltd.
P.O. Box 6651, Baulkham Hills, Business Centre, NSW 2153, Australia
Manufactured in the United States of America
Printed in Hong Kong
All rights reserved

Sterling ISBN 0-8069-8120-2

Contents

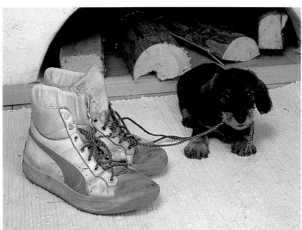

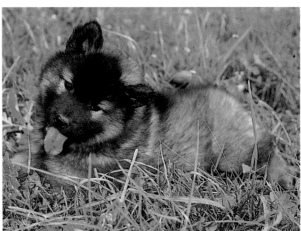

A pair of sneakers or warm grass—puppies have so much to explore.

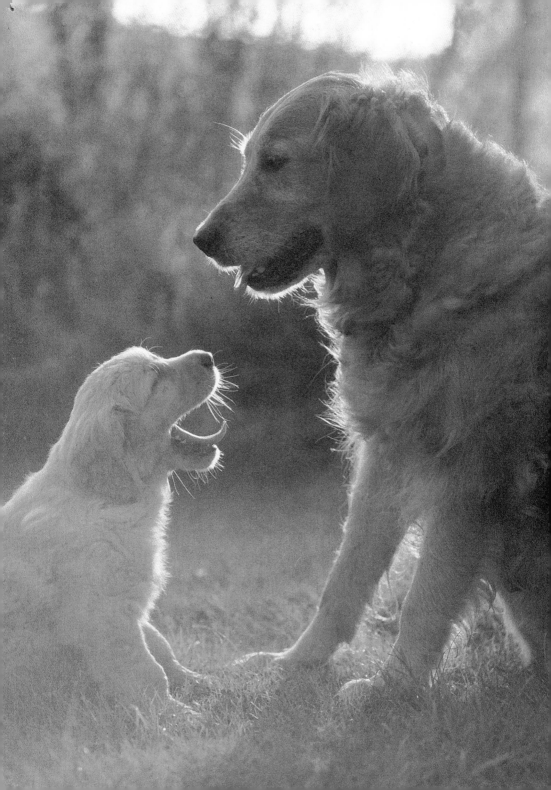

In this book, I want to give dog lovers information and tips on how to use natural healing methods to care for their sick pets. I'm not suggesting the use of natural methods as substitutes for or alternatives to conventional medicine; rather, I want dog lovers to use them as adjuncts to or extensions of conventional medicine. In general, a responsible nonmedical practitioner always works with a veterinarian, who will examine and treat any illnesses that are beyond the practitioner's capabilities. Sometimes, natural healing methods are a bit more time-consuming than the methods of allopathic (the use of drugs to alleviate symptoms) medicine, requiring more patience and commitment from the dog owner. The case histories from my practice make it clear that the necessary patience and commitment are worthwhile.

I always pay special attention to the affected organs or the injured part of the body when I design a therapy, but, as a nonmedical practitioner, I also take into consideration each dog's particular situation and environment. This may place extra demands on the owner, but one of the most important prerequisites for a healthy animal is an owner who is sensitive to its needs, including proper nutrition and proper handling.

Contact with its mother during the first ten to twelve weeks is vital for a puppy, assuring healthy physical and psychological development.

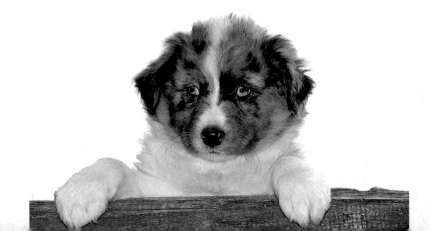

7

The Most Important Natural Healing Methods

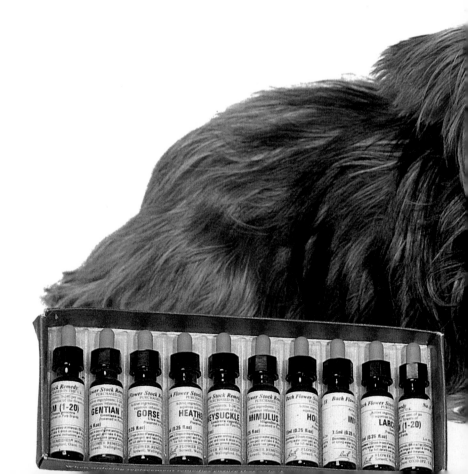

Natural Healing— What Is It?

Natural healing techniques teach us how to address health problems and injuries with natural methods. This is as true for animals as it is for people. Utilizing natural remedies means that we don't use chemical or pharmaceutical preparations; every remedy comes exclusively and directly from nature.

The different natural treatments known today are a combination of autonomous methods that should never be in conflict or competition with allopathic (the use of drugs to alleviate symptoms) medicine. Sometimes, the best interests of the patients may require using a combination of natural methods and conventional medicine.

Under no circumstances should you use natural methods hastily or indiscriminately. An accurate diagnosis is essential. For that reason, responsible practitioners use modern diagnostic methods, such as lab analysis of blood, stool, and urine, as well as X rays.

A natural practitioner will always try to treat the whole animal, including its

TIP

Many people believe that treatments using natural healing methods are tedious and time-consuming; this may or may not be the case. In many instances, these treatments achieve results in a surprisingly short period of time.

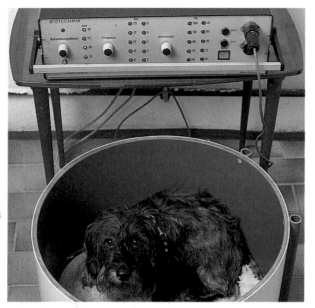

medicine for people, as well as for animals. The therapy consists of exposing diseased or injured parts of the body to an artificially created magnetic field for a few minutes. Scientists don't know yet how magnetic field therapy actually works. However, using a specific photo technique, researchers have noticed that when they expose an affected area to a small electrical energy flow, the temperature and flow of blood in that area increase, which in turn increases the oxygen available in the tissue.

We usually use magnetic field therapy for chronic inflammation, as well as for all degenerative bone and joint problems related to age or injuries.

The magnetic field surrounding Earth is a natural phenomenon. Electrical energy, or more precisely, the movement or flow of electrical energy can create a magnetic field artificially. Among other things, the strength or magnitude of such a magnetic field depends on the prevailing electrical current. Depending on the illness, the practitioner will treat the patient in a field of relatively higher or lower magnetic strength.

psychological state, and not just the symptoms. When you bring an injured dog into the office, a practioner will be just as concerned about the psychological shock the animal might have suffered as he or she will be about the injury and the physical condition.

But used exclusively, natural healing methods do have their limitations, for example, when the patient has lost its capacity for self-healing, when essential life-sustaining functions (such as insulin production) have stopped, or when optimum healing can only occur with surgery. In such cases, the patient should see a veterinarian.

Magnetic Field Therapy

Magnetic field therapy is a proven healing method often used in conventional

Leeches

The medicinal leech (*Hirudo medivinalis*), up to 6in (15cm) long, has a sucking organ on both ends. it attaches itself to the animal, bites through the skin, and sucks blood. Depending on its size, a leech can suck ½ teaspoon to 4 teaspoons (2 to 20ml) of blood, which it stores in its expandable stomach.

Natural practitioners use leeches raised specifically for medicinal purposes. The practitioner places them on the patient. When they have had their fill, they fall off by themselves. Afterwards, the area may bleed slightly for several hours, but it doesn't need to be covered.

The therapeutic effect is at least partially due to the decrease in the volume of blood in that specific area; the leeches' meal is a kind of bloodletting. In addition, the leeches' saliva, transferred to

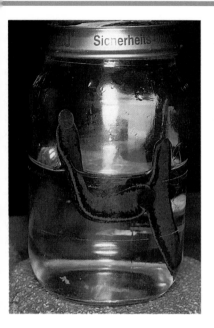

Founded at the end of the eighteenth century by Dr. Samuel Hahnemann (1755–1834), homeopathy means "healing with like." The basic principle states that whatever is making an organism sick can also heal it. According to this "law of similarity," you treat a patient with a medication containing an extremely diluted dose of a substance that, given in high doses, would cause an illness similar to what the patient has. On first thought, this seems rather paradoxical, but it works. Adherents believe that homeopathic medications activate an organism's own capacity for healing and that medications need to be geared very specifically to the illness.

In homeopathy, the term for this process is not "diluting the substances," but "increasing their potency." Supporters believe that during the production process, these substances go through a process of transformation. For instance, in order to produce a solution of Arnica 6 ×, you mix one drop of arnica tincture in a bottle with nine drops of alcohol and shake it ten times. You take one drop of the resulting solution in that bottle, called Arnica 1 ×, and mix it with nine drops of alcohol and shake it ten times. The result is Arnica 2 ×. In order to produce a 6 × formula, you must repeat the same procedure in the same manner, using the same proportions, four more times. Since every individual step thins a solution by a factor of ten, the amount of the original substance in the final mixture is unbelievably small. Preparing a 12 × formula, for instance, is much like putting one drop of a substance in a big lake and then filling a bottle with water from the lake. Nevertheless, a 12 × medication can be extremely effective. Shaking the substances at every step makes the difference.

Leeches live in shallow, stagnant bodies of water. However, leeches used by practitioners and veterinarian are raised in laboratories and shipped on demand.

TIP

The art of homeopathy consists of choosing the proper medication and knowing the proper doses. A homeopathic physician must be able to understand an illness in all its complexity, which in the case of an animal is even more complicated since the patient can't talk. For that reason, dog owners should refrain from treating their sick animals themselves. Instead, they should consult a licensed practitioner.

the patient's skin, contains substances that act as a local anesthetic and increase the circulation and coagulation of the blood. The application of leeches can often bring astounding results. For instance, when the patient suffers from arthritis and circulation problems, the improvement usually begins within twelve hours after the treatment.

Homeopathy

Many people think that homeopathy, one of the best-known forms of alternative healing, is the same as natural healing. However, homeopathy is only one of the methods used, even if it is one of the most prominent.

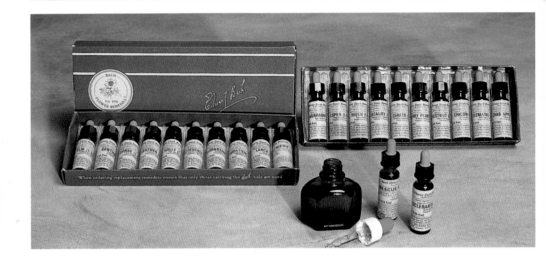

Used as drops, Bach flower remedies come in small bottles. Some of the flowers need to be collected on particular days and at particular times of the day and then prepared according to specific instructions.

Practitioners give homeopathic medications in the form of injections. They also suspend the medications in alcohol and use them in drops. In addition, they use them in small pear-shaped pellets made from milk sugar and a prepared solution. Homeopathic medications also come in salve form.

Mobilization Therapy

Practitioners often use mobilization therapy for chronic illnesses, particularly those of the skin, in which the body has lost its capacity to recognize illness. The result is that the body fails to make any attempt to heal itself. The therapy involves injecting a highly diluted pathogen, similar to the one that has caused the illness, into the body. Hopefully, this will stimulate the body to heal itself by mobilizing against the new attack and against the original illness.

Because this procedure puts a great deal of stress on the entire immune system, the patient's treatment should include measures that support the immune system.

Bach Flower Therapy

This therapy is the most controversial and the least accepted form of treatment among medical professionals. Dr. Edward Bach, a British physician, created the therapy in the early 1900s. He believed that every organic illness also has a psychological component. According to his hypothesis, if you remove the psychological problem, the organic symptoms will also go away. After decades of studying many, many plants and after conducting countless experiments on himself, he was able to rank 38 "flowers" according to their effects on different psychological symptoms and behaviors.

Bach flower preparations are made from whole flowers or parts of flowers and used as drops. Bach flower therapy is truly an art, requiring extensive education and training to choose the right combination of flowers for each individual medication.

Bach flower therapy depends entirely on experience. Scientists have found no explanation for how these flowers work or why no other combination can bring about the same results. However, experience has shown that in cases of shock and of difficulties in adjusting to new situations, this therapy produces astonishing results.

Compresses and Poultices

A poultice is nothing more than a simple, usually single-layered compress placed on an injured or painful part of the body. Of course, in real life this creates a problem because our patients seldom stand still for very long. You can use wet or dry compresses, and in many cases alternate both. You can also soak wet compresses in medical solutions or herbal teas.

As a general rule you use cold, wet compresses for acute inflammation. For almost all other conditions, use warm, wet compresses. You usually use dry and warm compresses for prolonged therapies. An ice bag is an example of a dry, cold compress. Only use a cold compress for a short time, about five minutes. You might leave a warm, dry compress in place for fifteen minutes.

Since compresses and poultices should provide comfort for the patient, use them gently and without force.

Organ Therapy

Although widely accepted in professional circles, this form of therapy is not well known among the lay population. It is somewhat similar to mobilization therapy, but the substances that go into the medication are unusual, for instance, colon bacteria (*Escherichia coli*), pyogenic organisms (*Staphylococcus aureus*), decaying meat (*Pyrogenia*), and certain organ tissues. The therapy involves injecting these substances, suspended in homeopathically prepared medications of different strengths, into the patient. While a great uncertainty exists about the way this method works, the applicability is very great. Some practitioners have achieved astounding results, particularly in cases of arthritis.

Autotransfusion

Since this method calls for taking blood from the patient, practitioners don't use it very often on small animals. In cases where the patient's own defense mechanism needs to be mobilized, the practitioner takes a small amount of blood from the patient and then immediately injects it in a muscle. In special cases, the practitioner may add oxygen to the

TIP

Many of the compresses that we use on ourselves we can also use on animals. You can find more detailed information in "Nursing Care," pages 78 to 92.

Calendula (orange marigold flowers) and chamomile flowers are surely two of the most well-known and most useful healing herbs. Borage (blue flowers) is useful for injuries; garlic is effective when used internally and for skin problems; and dried blueberries are very helpful in cases of diarrhea.

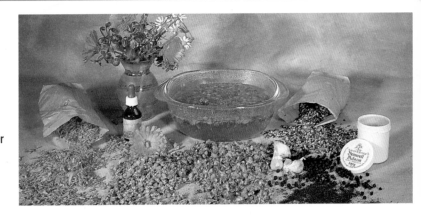

blood, use ultraviolet rays on the blood, or use a medication to fortify the blood before injecting it back into the patient. If, on the other hand, the practitioner wants to lower the patient's immune system, he removes a larger amount of blood. He makes the decision to reinject part of the withdrawn blood on a case-by-case basis. Taking larger amounts of blood often serves to relieve stress on the heart. In such cases, the practitioner doesn't return the blood to the patient's body.

Herbal Therapy

In its basic form, herbal therapy is surely one of the oldest healing methods in medicine. Herbal therapy makes use of the healing properties of plants. Since nature's garden has an herb for every illness, you can use herbal therapy in almost all cases. This is especially true because you can use numerous healing plants in many different ways and for many different situations. For instance,

you may take chamomile orally, but you can also use it for compresses and for inhalations. You can inject chamomile extract or use it in a healing salve.

Ozone Therapy

Ozone, a particular kind of oxygen, is a gas that has strong oxidation properties and changes easily into "normal" oxygen. In high concentrations, ozone has a very strong odor and is very poisonous. For treatment purposes, we use ozone in several different ways. One is to expose certain parts of the body to the gas, for example, in the treatment of persistent infections of mites to kill the parasites. We also use this therapy to treat blood that we have extracted before reinjecting it into the patient. This increases the body's own defense mechanism (see "Autotransfusion," page 13) and helps combat viral infections. To make use of the antibacterial property of ozone, we can also add it to olive oil to help treat wounds that are difficult to heal.

Acupuncture

This ancient Chinese healing method assumes that an imbalance in the flow of energy influences or causes every illness afflicting an organism. By stimulating very precise points (the acupuncture points) through the skin, the practitioner can reestablish the normal flow of energy. The classical form of acupuncture uses very thin needles made from silver or gold. Recently, acupuncturists have begun to use a laser beam instead of needles. They also use acupuncture points as sites for injecting medications, vitamins, and enzyme preparations.

Acupuncture can be helpful in many different conditions, including illnesses affecting internal organs, the blood, and the nervous system. In addition, an experienced acupuncturist can eliminate pain so completely that he can perform operations without anesthesia.

To know and be able to use the countless specific acupuncture points precisely during treatment is a high art. In large measure, success depends on the expertise and experience of the acupuncturist. Since the training and education for this healing art is very long and involved, only a few practitioners use acupuncture, and the ones who do usually use it only in uncomplicated cases.

The drawing shows the most important acupuncture points for dogs. When you stimulate these points with thin needles similar to those used in classical Chinese acupuncture, you can influence the functioning of the internal organs. Some practioners use a laser beam instead of needles.

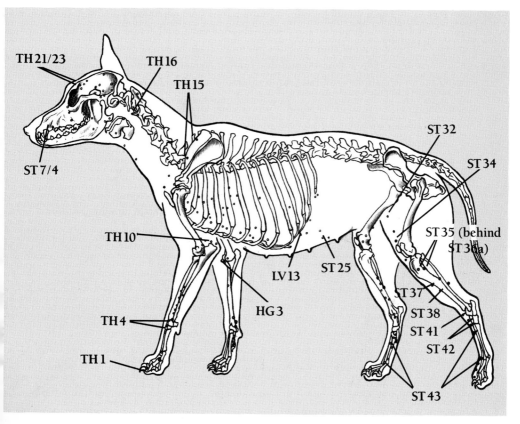

TIP

Do not treat your dog with herbs without establishing a proper diagnosis and without discussing the situation with you veterinarian or practitioner.

What follows is a list of medications and other aids that you ought to have on hand at all times. These medications make it possible for you to treat small discomforts and small injuries at home.

1. Medication

NOTE: Five drops are the equivalent of one tablet or five or six pellets. You can purchase medications and salves at health-food stores.

Apis 4 ×
Homeopathic medication made from bee venom. In case of an allergic reaction to an insect bite, give one tablet every ten minutes.

Arnica
As a diluted solution (arnica tincture in 1:100 ratio diluted in water) or as a salve for compresses in case of all nonbleeding injuries, such as strains and sprains.

At a strength of 4 × or 6 ×, a homeopathic remedy for any injury: give five drops every hour until symptoms improve, then three times a day.

Blueberry (dried form)
As a powder, mixed into food. Brings quick and effective relief from diarrhea.

Borage
Use in the form of compresses for every type of injury. Helps to stop bleeding and inflammation. For a compress, boil 3½oz (100g) of borage roots in 1qt (1l) of water for ten minutes.

Natural Healing Remedies

Calendula (common or pot marigold)
Used as a medicine for almost everything that ails us and our dogs.

As an oil, for the treatment of ear mites and ear infections. As a diluted solution from a tincture, for insect bites or ear infections. As a tea, for inhalation for respiratory problems. As a salve, for small injuries.

Chamomile
As a tea, for stomach and intestinal problems and for inhalations in cases of respiratory problems.

Added to the bath, for skin problems.

As a diluted solution from tincture, used for compresses for poorly healing wounds.

Coltsfoot
As a tea (using the flowers as well as the leaves), for inhalation for respiratory problems. As an expectorant, has infection-fighting properties. The tea relieves many types of coughs when used for inhalation several times a day.

Echinacea
Made from the *Echinacea angustifolia* flower, which grows wild in North America.

As a salve, for wounds that won't heal.

As drops, for infectious diseases and to stimulate the body's own healing power.

Garlic
In tablet form, granules, or crushed cloves, add to food. Effective against all parasitic, fungal, and skin dis-

...ases. (Garlic is not a substitute for regular treatment against worms!)

Healing Earth
Can buy ready-made for oral application for intestinal problems. Used externally as a compress or as an additive to the bath.

Indian Nerve Tea
Can buy ready-made to mix with food.

Kaopectate
As a liquid, a ready-made preparation for diarrhea. Give your dog ½ to 2 teaspoons (2 to 10ml), depending on weight, up to five times a day.

Nux vomica 6 ×
A homeopathic medication used to control vomiting. Start with one tablet every hour, then try two tablets three times a day.

Important: Do not give to a pregnant dog.

Paraffin Oil
Clear oil made from the residues of oil-refining process. Often used as a base for salves. For constipation, mix approximately ½ teaspoon (2ml) in with food.

Peppermint
As a tea, for inhalation for respiratory problems and as a drink for stomach problems.

Rescue Remedy
As drops, a Bach flower remedy for any type of shock. Give three drops every five minutes. Can also apply to the skin. Best place to apply is between the ears.

Traumeel
As a tablet, for any kind of injury. Give several times during the day. Consists of several different homeopathic remedies and *Echinacea*.

Varatrum album 4 ×
A homeopathic medication made from sprouted wheat, a plant belonging to the lily family that grows in the Alps. In North America the variety is known as American white hellebore, *Veratum viride*.

Stimulates the circulatory system.

As a tablet, for acute failure of the circulatory system. Give one tablet (best if crushed), repeat after ten minutes.

2. Other Aids

A thermometer, scissors, elastic, plastic and tube bandages, disinfectant

A cotton blanket and a wool sock from which the tip has been cut off to use as a compress

Several disposable syringes (without the needles) to hold ½ teaspoon (2ml) and 4 teaspoons (20ml) to administer teas and other liquid medications

A blanket or other piece of cloth to keep the animal warm or to transport a severely injured or very sick animal; also used as an aid during the treatment of particularly difficult patients

A hot-water bottle or electric heating pad

TIP

In cases of discomfort or illness, always support the therapy with an appropriate diet (see "Diets in Cases of Illnesses").

17

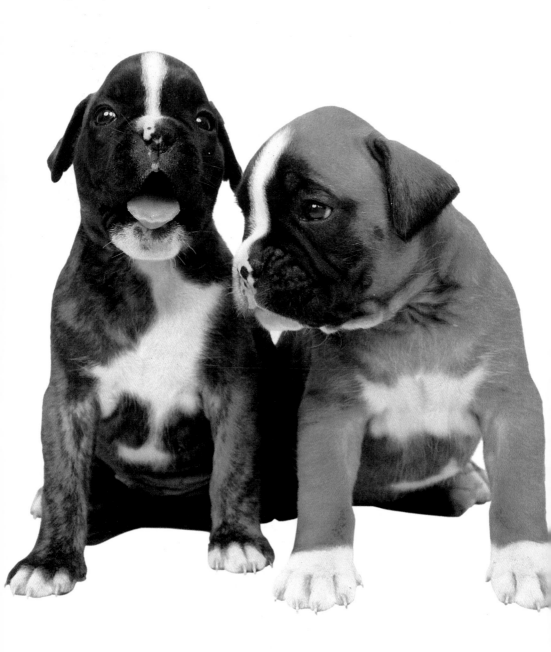

Developmental Stages of a Young Dog

Who can resist watching the antics of a young puppy exploring its world with its big paws and even bigger tummy? Most people find that they can't be angry with these little creatures even if, as is the case with "children," they get themselves in all sorts of trouble during their exploratory phase and later when they are adolescents. To create a harmonious union between man and dog, a puppy needs human contact and consistent training very early in its life.

From Birth to the Third Week

A dog's pregnancy usually lasts sixty-three days; but just as with humans, variations of a few days either way are normal.

At birth, puppies are deaf and blind and their sense of smell is not yet fully developed. They can only find their mother's nipples by using their innate searching instinct. At birth, the only significantly developed sense is the sense of taste.

When the mother is not there, puppies always huddle close together, often sleeping on top of each other. This is a good way for them to keep warm because they lack the ability to maintain a constant body temperature over an extended period of time. In the case of a single birth, the puppy is very much at a disadvantage and needs a heating pad to stay warm (see "Nursing Care," page 88).

In the beginning, a puppy's day consists entirely of nursing and sleeping. The mother will lick the puppy's stomach and rectal areas in order to stimulate digestion and the excretion of stool and urine. Without this stimulation, a puppy is incapable of producing either.

19

Top: Healthy newborn puppies find their mother's nipples relatively quickly. The first milk that the mother dog produces contains important immunity-producing substances that provide protection against infectious diseases.

Left: Drinking and sleeping are the only activities of newborn puppies. They sleep huddled together to keep themselves warm.

Right: When they are about four weeks old, puppies begin serious play. They fiercely protect their toys from their siblings. Biting into a rubber ball encourages the appearance of first teeth, which occurs between the third and fifth weeks of life.

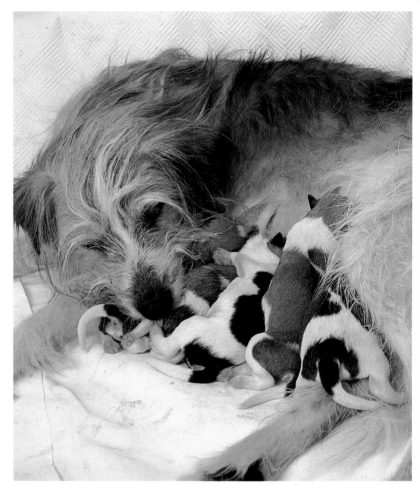

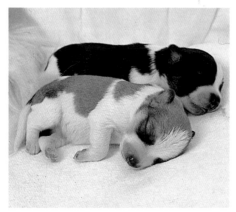

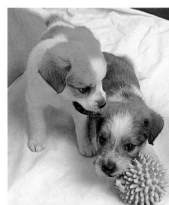

In order to keep the "nursery" clean, the mother very carefully licks up all discharges. Puppies begin opening their eyes when they are about one week old. The first sign is a small slit at the inside corner of the eyes. The eyes open completely during the course of the next two to three days. However, a puppy's vision isn't fully developed for several weeks. The sense of hearing and the sense of smell also develop slowly. They are fully developed by the time the puppy is four weeks old.

The initial attempts to stand up and walk start as early as the first week. Most of the time, however, these attempts amount to no more than a crawl because both the head the full tummy are too heavy. By the second week, puppies start to explore their immediate environment, even if their legs are still rather wobbly. At the same time, they begin to push and bite their siblings, and now and then you can hear little growls and something that sounds like a bark. When their teeth begin to erupt, puppies will chew on anything they find.

At this stage, their mother is still the only source of nutrition, warmth, and security. She is the center of their world. Most female dogs are devoted mothers, but even devoted mothers may give a little growl when their puppies are nursing too eagerly. If a mother dog is not available or simply does not care for her young, you must provide a "wet nurse" for the puppies. Puppies should only be bottle-fed for a short period of time. For the first eight to twelve weeks, the presence of a mother dog is absolutely essential for the young puppies, improving their changes of survival. Bottle-fed puppies are in much more danger than those raised by a mother dog. A female dog that serves as "wet nurse" should be about the same size as the mother of the puppies. She should also be the same breed (or a similar breed) as the puppies and should have no more than five puppies of her own. Her own puppies should not be more than ten days older or younger than the orphaned or neglected puppies.

Ask your veterinarian or practitioner what you need to know until you can find a substitute mother for your puppies. Because of the enormous differences in the size of different breeds, specific information about the proper amount of food is difficult to give. What is most important is that the puppies continue to gain weight, and this means that you must weigh them daily.

Fourth to Eighth Week

Now your puppies are very active. They are busy exploring their environment, venturing farther and farther from their

Even if their legs are still somewhat wobbly, three-week-old puppies begin to explore their environment.

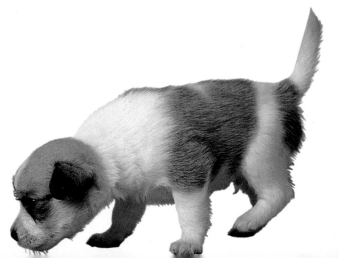

TIP

If you need to find a substitute mother to be a "wet nurse" for your puppies, ask your veterinarian or practitioner for help. They may know of a dog that has recently given birth. Place advertisements in your local newspaper and check with dog clubs. Local radio stations may be willing to help, too.

Nutritional Information

First Feedings

- Begin offering puppies solid food when they are four weeks old. The food should be available to them throughout the day.
- When they are eight weeks old, feed them approximately six times a day.
- Until puberty, feed them three to four times a day.
- After puberty, feed them once or twice a day.

First Foods

Most puppies do well on commercial puppy food (wet or dry) and on oats soaked in water. Rapidly growing puppies need additional calcium.

Weight Gain

Puppies need to increase their weight every day. The exact amount of the weight gain depends on the breed. Check with your veterinarian or practitioner. You need to weigh them once a week if their mother is feeding them, but you'll need to check daily if you are bottle-feeding them. Lack of weight gain is a symptom of other problems. You'll need to consult your veterinarian or practitioner as quickly as possible.

Supplemental Feeding

If the litter contains more than six puppies, you may have to give them additonal food. Supplemental feedings might also be necessary for puppies delivered by Cesarean section or whose mother becomes sick and cannot nurse them. If the puppies are still nursing, you'll need to bottle-feed them. (Special feeding bottles with the appropriate nipple are available at pet stores.) Later, you may give them oatmeal from a plate or let them lick it off your fingers.

Give additional food to the biggest puppies so that their smaller siblings get more of their mother's milk, always the best nutrition. If necessary, you may offer additional food to a particularly small puppy. You can support normal and healthy development and stimulate the immune system for even the smallest and weakest of the litter if you use vitamins and other natural supplements. Consult your practitioner for specifics. (You'll find information on a therapy that helps strengthen weak puppies on page 32 under "Case Histories.")

If necessary, you can give a puppy a mixture of semisolid and solid food as early as the third week. Pureed boiled beef mixed with rice and carrots and some vegetables works very well. You can also give puppies baby foods with meat and vegetables as long as they have no gluten, dairy products, salt, or sugar. Offer this from a plate or use a disposable syringe, dripping the food gently into the mouth. Puppies have a period of adjustment when they go from their mother's milk to solid food. They may have slight diarrhea during this period. In most cases a little cottage cheese or pureed carrots takes care of the problem. (See "The Most Frequently Occurring Illnesses, pages 30 and 31.)

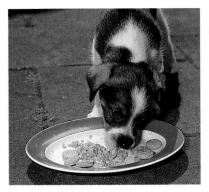

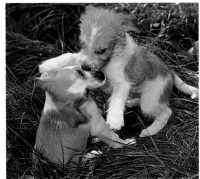

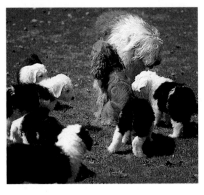

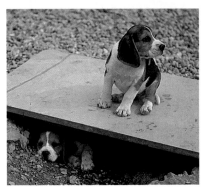

Top left: This five-week-old puppy is slurping his puppy cereal and munching on his first dog biscuit.

Top right: Playing with siblings is very important for healthy psychological development.

Below left: A male cocker spaniel being checked out by a curious bobtail puppy isn't very happy. In fact, his body language conveys fear.

Below right: These nine-week-old puppies are investigating every corner of their environment. They no longer need to be near their mother.

mother. They want to check out everything new they encounter. Depending on their temperment, they are very attentive, but only from a safe distance. Their sense of hearing and sense of smell are now fully developed. During warm, dry days, puppies love to be outside for hours at a time, but the family needs a dry place, protected from the wind. This is where the puppies will rest and nurse.

Even at this tender age, personalities begin to form. As you watch them play, you'll notice that a certain order of dominance is beginning to emerge.

The puppies now deposit their urine and stool without assistance, and the mother won't remove it anymore. You'll need to be sure that their living area is accessible so that you can clean it easily.

Ninth to Twelfth Week

The puppies are more and more independent and venture farther and farther away from the mother, She will still keep a watchful eye on her brood, but she also gives them more freedom to explore. The puppies become less and less interested in their mother's milk, and their mother will begin to push them away with a growl. This completes the process of weaning, begun when you introduced the puppies to solid food, and the mother's milk dries up. At the same time as they are becoming physically independent of their mother, puppies are also becoming increasingly psychologically independent. This is the time when a puppy wants the companionship of humans. Although timing varies from breed to breed, in general this takes place around the tenth week.

At this stage in the development of their socialization, they need someone to be consistently involved with them. The experiences they have now, good or bad, loving or thoughtless, influence their character for the rest of their lives.

When your puppy is eight weeks old, you must have it immunized. Since every immunization takes its toll on the whole organism, the animal should be very healthy, active, and already dewormed. The following discusses the type of protective immunization a dog needs and when you need to deworm it.

Immunization and Deworming Schedule

Four, Six, and Eight Weeks Old
Deworming

Eight Weeks Old
After deworming, basic immunization against distemper, infectious liver inflammation, and leptospirosis (one injection); also against parvo virus infection

Twelve Weeks Old
Deworming
After deworming, second basic immunizations as above; in addition, against rabies

Danger of Infection!

During the period when puppies are beginning to eat solid food, they are also seriously investigating their environment. As a result, they come in very close contact with germs in their environment. Since their mother's milk provides very little in the way of protection, young dogs are in danger of contracting infectious diseases.

If a puppy shows any signs of discomfort, including reduced food intake, apathy, diarrhea or vomiting, take its temperature. You'll find suggestions on how to do that in "Nursing Care," page 78.

If the puppy's temperature is above 102.5°F (39.3°C) or below 100.5°F (38°C), see your veterinarian immediately. If the temperature is normal, between 100.5°F (38°C) and 102°F (39°C), a telephone call might be all that is necessary. You can find information about natural home remedies in the table "The Most Frequently Occurring Illnesses," pages 30 and 31, and in a list of natural remedies in the medicine cabinet, pages 16 and 17.

Of course, if the puppy takes a turn for the worse or does not improve after twenty-four hours, take the puppy to your veterinarian immediately.

Six and Nine Months Old (then twice a year)
Deworming

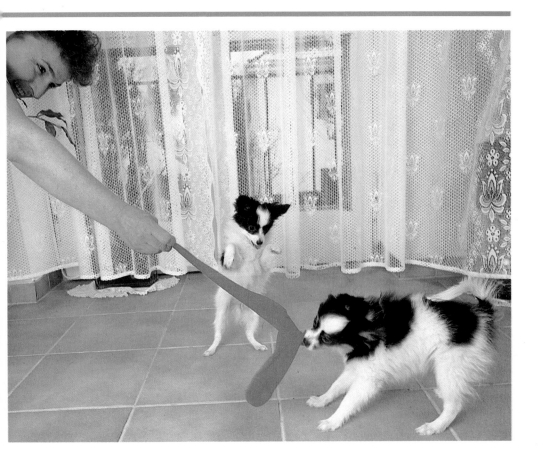

14 Months Old
Booster shots against all five infectious diseases

Every Year
Booster shots against leptospirosis, parvo virus infection, and rabies

Every Two Years
Booster shots against distemper and infectious liver inflammation

Now, playtime among the puppies is more boisterous and much louder. Their voices might still be puppylike, but they already have all of the typical vocal expressions of an adult dog. All play with human beings includes happy barking and the mother's warning bark. Her watchful bark provokes a playful puppy bark. Accompanied by scary-sounding growls, the little creatures tussle and fight to take possession of a prized prey (often simply a favorite toy).

The individual temperaments and characteristics of each puppy are now easy to identify. Some are fearless; others are easily frightened. Some are particularly clumsy; others are shy and careful. Such observations are important when it comes time to find the right home for each puppy.

Positive experiences with a human being help a puppy develop into a happy, socially well-adjusted family dog.

Above: Since young dogs relieve themselves frequently, a layer of newspaper on the floor is a good temporary solution. However, make sure that using the newspaper does not turn into a habit. Use it strictly as the first step in housebreaking.

Below: Lavish praise is an important part of training puppies because encouraging words and pats make learning fun for a puppy.

TIP

Don't send a puppy to its new home until it is no longer dependent on its mother and until it has become attached to humans.

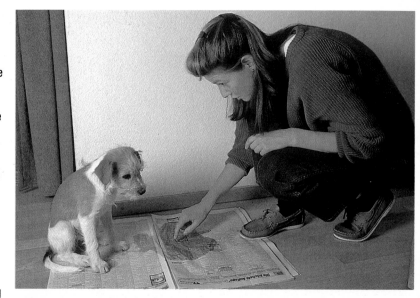

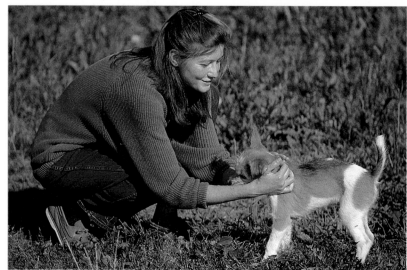

This brings us to the subject of saying goodbye. The proper time to give it to its new owner depends on the individual developmental stage of the puppy. While a strong, somewhat independent ten-week-old puppy may do fine when you place it with its new family, a weaker and less self-confident puppy would greatly profit if allowed to remain for another two weeks with its mother. By the end of twelve weeks, all puppies are ready to leave their mothers, and most puppies are independent enough to adjust to a new family.

Fourth to Sixth Month

In general, puppies have new homes by this age. This means that they not only have to get used to new smells and sounds but also to the existing family dynamics.

The first two weeks in a new environment determine the quality of the relationship between a puppy and the members of the family. As soon as a puppy has gotten the lay of the land, which usually takes no more than a couple of days, you should begin intensive training. Most important of all, you must teach the young dog to only relieve itself *outside,* and then, only where permitted. In addition, you have to teach the dog to "give notice" when it feels the urge. In the beginning, you'll need to take your dog outside after each meal or after a long nap. Give the dog lavish praise after it has completed its "business." Praise provides excellent reinforcement and assures the dog that it is doing well. Naturally, it will then want to repeat the behavior. Always try to bring the dog to a spot that other dogs have used. You'll also need to get up during the night as soon as the puppy gets restless. This is inconvenient but is only necessary for four weeks. After that time, the dog will be housebroken.

You should never reprimand or hit a dog after it has had an accident indoors, because the dog is not capable of making the connection between the accident, which might have happened some time ago, and the punishment. Only voice disapproval if you actually witness the accident—because at that point, the dog

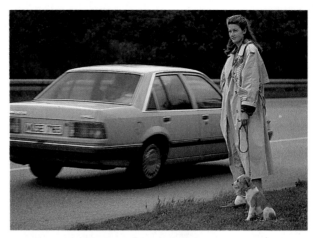

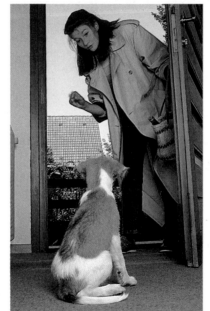

Above: A dog should automatically sit when it nears a curb.

Left: Dogs should never be left alone for more than four to five hours. But they must learn to be by themselves. Start leaving them alone for short periods of about five minutes and slowly extend the time.

will be able to connect the accident and your reprimand.

But housebreaking is not the end of training. You'll also want to teach your dog to behave properly on a leash and to promptly follow commands such as "Sit," "Stay," and "Down." The subject of

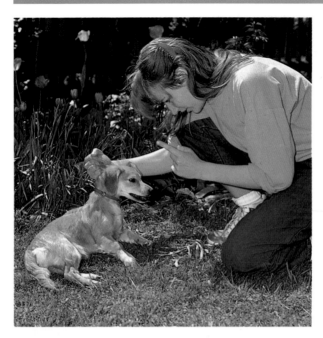

words. Always reprimand or punish the dog immediately after the misbehavior occurs, so that your dog can make the connection between the deed and the consequences. Screaming and hitting a disobedient dog is useless because all the dog learns is to be afraid.

Seventh to Twelfth Month

This is the period of adolescence and mischief called puberty. During this time, male dogs are particularly rebellious, not unlike their human counterparts. With great determination, a young dog will attempt to improve his rank in the "pack." At times you may think that he has forgotten everything that he ever learned, including all of the commands. Sometimes he may even growl at you. He is obviously trying to challenge your status as the "head of the pack." Your dog will only accept his place if you demand unquestioned obedience during this period. If you don't, he may well develop into a real tyrant.

Contact with other male dogs can quickly turn into fights (including biting) during this phase. However, you should encourage contact with the female members of his species because this interaction is vital for the healthy psychological development of a dog.

During this period your dog will also go through a lot of external changes. Weight gain slows down dramatically, the body becomes longer, the dog loses its puppylike clumsiness and begins to grow into the proportions of an adult

Punishing your dog only makes sense when you catch your dog immediately after the misdeed. Grab the dog's neck and give a short shake. This is a clear sign to the dog that it has misbehaved, because it is the same method that its mother used when she corrected one of her puppies.

dog training is too broad to discuss in this book, but we'll take a look at a few basic rules that are absolutely essential for a healthy, long-term relationship between you and your dog.

One of the most important elements for successful training and obedience is consistently demanding that *your* will prevails at all times. If you give clear and consistent commands in the same tone of voice, the dog will understand what you expect.

If you allow your dog to ignore the "Sit" command today, you should not be surprised if the dog ignores the same command tomorrow.

You'll need to praise your dog with more than just words. A friendly pat on the back, stroking behind the ears, and even a little treat will go a long way towards making training sessions fun. Reprimands should be unambiguous. Use a sharp tone of voice and the same

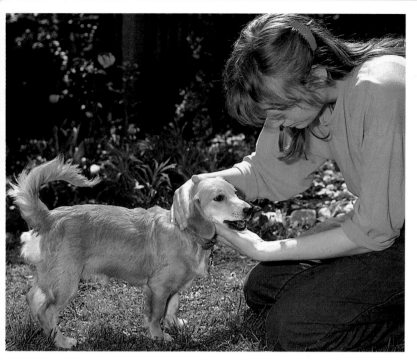

Positive reinforcement is very important. If your dog has been obeying your commands, use pats and praises to reinforce the commands.

TIP

Try not to go on vacation for the first few months after your dog comes to live with you. Being left without you is psychologically stressful, and your dog may become susceptible to infectious diseases.

Growing Permanent Teeth

During this period, young dogs have to cope with the loss of their "milk" teeth and the eruption of their permanent ones. Teething usually starts during the fifth month and is over between the sixth and eighth month. It is a painful process because the gums are often swollen and may become infected. Many dogs stop eating for a couple of days. Some experience a considerable increase in the flow of saliva, and sometimes they even vomit. Other dogs try to get relief by constantly chewing on hard objects. If your dog's "milk" teeth don't fall out by themselves, you'll need your veterinarian's help.

dog. The voice becomes deeper, and the bark begins to sound much more like that of an adult dog. At about the age of seven months, a male dog begins to lift his leg when urinating. Many female dogs come into heat for the first time at this age.

When they are about one year old, most dogs have completed adolescence. The young dog is now an adult.

TIP

Make sure that the smaller and less assertive puppies get enough to eat. If the puppies vary significantly in size, weight, and temperaments, serve food in several dishes. Feed small puppies at least three times a day. Take the mother out of the room or for a walk while the puppies are eating.

The Most Frequentl

Recognizable Symptoms	Possible Reasons
Yellow or watery discharge from the eyes; swollen or sticky eyelids	Conjunctivitis or common illness, such as distemper; or genetic eye problem
Constant watery yellow discharge from the nose, loud breathing, or frequent sneezing	Common illness, such as distemper; bacterial infection of the upper respiratory tract; foreign object in the nose
Black, sticky layer inside the ears; constantly shaking the head (itching); won't tolerate touch	Parasites; foreign object inside; ears plugged up; dirt or dried blood inside; bacterial infection or bleeding from ear (particularly with long-eared dogs)
Black or white objects attached to the fur; bare spots with or without scabs; frequent or incessant scratching (itching)	Skin parasites such as lice, fleas, skin mites; skin fungus or allergies
Swelling under the skin; abscess	Intestinal parasites such as in spool worm, hookworm, or to rectum; tapeworm; bacterial infection of intestinal tract, such as distemper or parvo virus (unlikely)
Swollen stomach; loud noises the intestines; stool sticking; dog drags its behind over the ground; discharge from the genitalia	Vaginitis or prepuce infection; symptoms as part of distemper
Loss of appetite or constant hunger, but losing weight	Parasite infestation of the intestinal tract; chronic illness of the pancreas
Lame; joints sensitive to the touch	Sprain or bruise; injury to the ligaments or other injuries; joints congenitally misshapen
Sudden loss of appetite and apathy	Beginning of infectious parasite disease; parasite infection of internal organs; poisoning; swallowed foreign object
Diarrhea and intestinal tract	Viral infection; poisoning; parasite infection of the stomach
Vomiting	Viral infection; inflammation of the stomach lining; poisoning; swallowed foreign object; parasite infection of the stomach and intestinal tract

ccurring Illnesses

What You Can Do	See Your Veterinarian If
ke temperature; watch for other symptoms; cool mpresses with diluted chamomile tea; give *Euphrasia* × several times a day	No improvement within three days; you cannot rule out the presence of a foreign object or injury; additional symptoms appear, such as temperature above 102.5°F (39.3°C) or below 100.5°F (38°C)
ke temperature; inhalation therapy using chamomile; ply salve	No improvement within three days; symptoms get worse; additional symptoms appear, such as vomiting or apathy; temperature above 102.5°F (39.3°C) or below 100.5°F (38°C); you cannot rule out the presence of a foreign object
e ozone-enriched olive oil or calendula oil in the ears	You suspect a foreign object; extreme sensitivity to touch or swollen; no improvement within five days
eat with flea powder or bathe with citronella; give enty of garlic (also in the form of tablets); Traumeel blets	Cannot detect parasites; severe skin inflammation has developed
ve *Myristica sebifera* 6 × to bring an abscess to a ad, use *hepar sulfuris* 8 ×; to heal an abscess, use epar sulfuris 12 ×	Abscess is large
worm and repeat on schedule in the future; take mperature; observe closely and pay attention to ditional signs of illness	No improvement within three days; additional symptoms appear, including temperature above 102.5°F (39.3°C) or below 100.5°F (38°C)
ve preparation to support the body's own healing wer such as *Echinacea*; wash with chamomile or lendula tea	No improvement within one week; additional symptoms appear
worm and repeat on schedule in the future; give garlic d vitamin B; in case of flatulance add fennel, anise, d caraway seeds	Parasites or a pancreatic infection is present; both always require treatment
ply ice bag or arnica compress; give *Traumeel* medica- on in short intervals; check carefully for injuries; keep alks to a minimum	Animal cannot use or move a leg or paw; is afraid of touch; bone seems displaced; large wounds are present; foreign objects embedded; no improvement within three days
ke temperature; observe closely; give *Echinacea*; avoid citement and stress; keep walks to a minimum	Temperature above 102.5°F (39.3°C) or below 100.5°F (38°C); no improvement within three days; other symptoms appear
ke temperature; give only chamomile and weak black a for twenty-four hours, then only a light diet (fish, cken, rice); keep close watch; give charcoal and hinacea several times daily	No obvious improvement for several days; other symptoms appear; poisoning seems possible; temperature above 102.5°F (39.3°C) or below 100.5°F (38°C)

TIP

Between the ninth and twelfth months, your young dog needs to be thoroughly examined. The sooner a professional detects inherited problems or weaknesses, the sooner you can initiate the appropriate preventive or strengthening measures.

Case Histories from My Practice

How much a puppy should weigh depends on its breed, but whatever the breed, the puppy needs to gain weight consistently. You should weigh your puppy once a week and every day when it is sick.

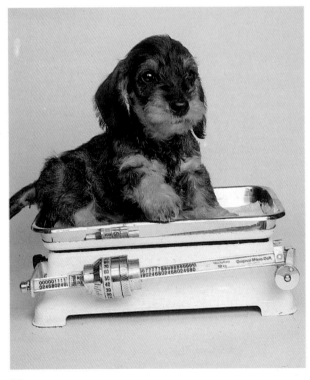

Constitution Therapy

Some puppies do not thrive. This is especially true of some that are part of a large litter. These puppies are weak and always seem to be behind in their development when compared to their stronger siblings. A vicious cycle often starts: the smaller puppy gets less milk because the other members of the litter keep pushing it away from the mother's nipples. The result is that the puppy gets even weaker and even less able to fight back. Not getting enough of its mother's milk also makes a puppy more susceptible to illnesses. Such a puppy, often called the runt of the litter, is much more likely to contract infectious diseases. If we do not intervene in time, the puppy may have a weak immune system for a long time, and its development will always lag behind that of its siblings.

Coco, a five-month-old male terrier, was just such a runt. His owner was constantly concerned for him. She had bought the dog in a pet shop because she felt sorry for him. His stronger and much more lively siblings had all found homes very quickly. He was the only one of his litter left in the shop. Coco had been sick almost constantly since he arrived in his new home. First he suffered from diarrhea, than angina, next from a bladder infection which resulted in prepuce infection. Antibiotics were only effective for a short period of time.

Through word of mouth, the owner had learned I was having good results using a special constitutional therapy in similar cases. Constitutional therapy strengthens and stabilizes the physical condition and resistance of weak puppies. Coco's owner contacted me and made an appointment.

Coco, whose weight was very low for his age, allowed me to examine him without any resistance. I found no signs of any grave or acute disease. After a long conversation with the owner about Coco's physical and psychological situation, I put together a treatment plan using high-potency homeopathic remedies and a combination of Bach flower remedies. In addition, I recommended a weekly vitamin supplement combined with a medication that would stimultate the dog's own immune system. I also included an enzyme preparation that would detoxify the body.

Coco's treatment lasted five weeks. By that time, he was gaining weight steadily, and no new infections had appeared. The change from milk teeth to permanent teeth that took place during this time created no problems for the little guy.

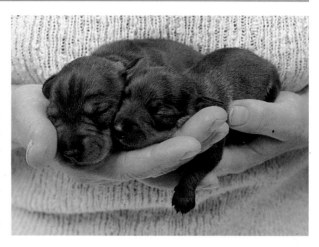

Nose and Throat Inflammations

Dogs can suffer from colds and sore throats just as people can. Although the germs are sometimes the same, people and animals don't usually infect each other. That was one thing that I could assure the owner when she came in with Tony, her five-month-old Labrador retriever. She was concerned about her dog and also about her two children and her cat. For the last couple of days, the patient had not been as lively as usual, and he was only eating very little.

When I examined Tony, I found that he had a slightly elevated temperature and an inflamed throat. I gave him an injection of a plant remedy in order to increase his own defense mechanism and a homeopathic remedy for his sore throat. I told the owner to give the same medication to her dog five to six times daily for the next several days. I also

Individual puppies from the same litter come in many different sizes, particularly in mixed breeds. Sometimes one of the puppies is very weak and needs special care and attention from the owner.

Above: From the fourth week on, puppies can play outside in nice weather. As they get older, their world expands.

Below: Puppies suffering from flower allergies might not have so much fun outside.

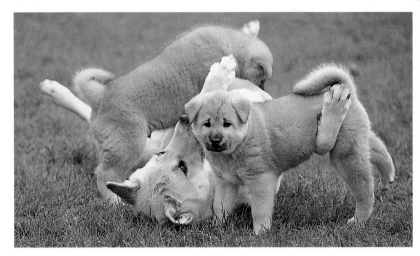

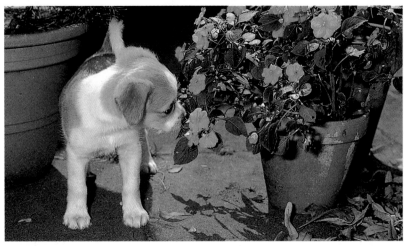

recommended that she put a wet, cold compress around the dog's neck twice a day to lower his temperature.

The owner came back two days later. The inflammation in the throat had improved markedly. I repeated the injection and provided the owner with another homeopathic medication that she was to give Tony three times a day for five days. When Tony came back five days later, all his symptoms had disappeared.

Pollen Allergies

Annoying allergies, such as hay fever, bother dogs, too. Dogs can have allergic reactions to grasses and all kinds of other plants. Just like people, their main symptoms are frequent sneezing, a runny nose, and itching eyes, often with a watery, clear discharge.

Dangerous Illnesses

Parvo virus is one of the most feared of all the illnesses that can infect puppies and adult dogs. It is a highly infectious viral disease passed from one dog to another. It can also be transmitted by people, by their clothes, and by other objects. The highly resistant virus can even survive outside of a host for many months. Very few disinfection methods work against it.

Although adult dogs are not immune to this virus, the vast majority of parvo virus patients are less than six months old. The incubation period, the time from the moment the infection enters the body until symptoms appear, is anywhere from one to seven days. The most prominent symptoms are diarrhea and vomiting. In many cases, the blood does not coagulate well, and the temperature is below normal. Death comes very quickly as a result of a general collapse of the circulatory system and of the heart. However, a dog who has survived the first three or four days is usually out of the woods and will be able to survive this insidious disease. Unfortunately, parvo virus often leaves the dog with heart and liver problems.

Distemper is a viral infection that is somewhat unpredictable, appearing in different forms and progressing in many different ways. In most cases, it leads to death. If the dog survives, it often has many health problems. Puppies and young dogs are in particular danger. The most common form is lung distemper, but the disease can also attack the throat and the bronchial area. Severe pneumonia sets in when the lungs are involved. Stomach and intestinal distemper attacks the mucus membranes of the stomach and the intestinal tract, leading to diarrhea and vomiting. Distemper of the central nervous system is especially feared. During the course of the illness, the dog experiences cramps, epileptic seizures, and paralysis. If the lungs are paralyzed, the dog's life comes to an abrupt end. Different forms of distemper can appear singly, in combination, or successively.

Infection inevitably occurs when a dog comes in contact with another infected dog, sniffs the stool or urine of such an animal, or sniffs and licks the infected animal, or vice versa. The illness is evident within three to seven days after the infection occurs, either violently with temperatures up to 105.5°F (41°C) or, more likely, with a harmless cold. Infected dogs can transmit the distemper virus for two months and are an ongoing source of the disease. Even a mother who appears to be perfectly healthy can transmit the virus to her puppies.

Regular immunizations can protect animals from both diseases. In my practice, I have treated parvo virus and distemper with great success. However, successful treatment depends on detecting the illness as early as possible.

TIP

Don't try to keep your dog away from other dogs because of your fear of infection. Contact with other dogs is a very important element in the psychological health of a dog. Just be sure that your dog receives the proper immunizations at the proper times.

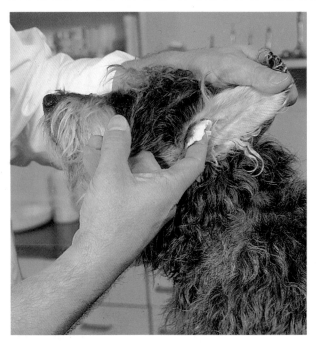

A week later, the owner reported that the puppy still had some reactions when he was outside for any length of time but that the reactions were much less severe.

I had to caution the owner that the danger of a distemper infection was still present. For that reason, I suggested that he watch the puppy closely and that he contact me immediately if the symptoms worsened or if new ones appeared.

Foreskin Infection

Inflammation of the foreskin, an inflammation of the soft tissue of the penis and foreskin, is common but harmless. Caused by bacteria and dirt in the foreskin, it occurs most often in dogs whose immune systems are not strong enough to fight infectious diseases.

His owner brought Rex, a five-year-old German shepherd, to my office with such an infection. A few weeks before, the dog had suffered from diarrhea, and now the infection was so severe that he needed professional help. The itching was so bad that the dog was licking his genitalia constantly.

When I examined Rex, I immediately noticed a thick yellow discharge dripping from around the opening of the foreskin, which made the diagnosis easy. I informed the owner of the diagnosis and told him that the primary reason for this infection was that the dog's immune system was very weak. I prescribed a medication consisting of several different plant extracts which would strengthen the immune system. In addition, I advised the owner to wash the dog's genitalia daily with a concentrated

Ear mites are parasites that may cause ear infections. But too much ear wax can also cause problems. To prevent problems, check your pet's ears regularly.

These were the symptoms described to me by Benno's owner one spring. Five-week-old Benno was let outside in the garden for the first time. In just a few minutes, he began to sneeze continuously. Soon his nose and eyes were dripping.

I examined him carefully to make sure that the little guy was not in the first stages of a dangerous viral infection, such as distemper. However, Benno seemed to be healthy and lively, but his eyes showed signs of conjunctivitis. I explained the connection to the owner and suggested that he leave the dog indoors while grasses were in bloom. In addition, I prescribed a natural salve as well as cool compresses for the eyes. We also attempted to lessen Benno's reaction to allergy-causing agents by giving him a specific enzyme preparation and a homeopathic medication.

solution of chamomile, arnica, and hamamelis. I also instructed him to apply *Echinacea* salve to the foreskin and the tip of the penis. The best way to do this is with a disposable syringe, without the needle, of course.

In only three days, Rex's improvement was noticeable, and within ten days all symptoms had disappeared.

Parasite Infection

Regular deworming and good hygiene are essential to protect your dog from parasite invasions. They are also necessary to cure parasite infections. If you ignore parasites, they can reproduce until the result is a massive infestation. Such was the case with Mona, a thirteen-week-old dog whose owner had brought her home from a vacation in Italy. The

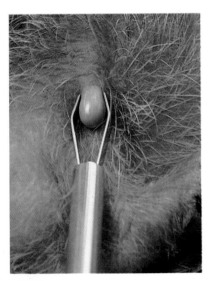

owner was very concerned because Mona had an enormous appetite which was never satisfied, and despite all the food she was eating, Mona was not gaining any weight. In addition to her constant hunger, the dog had a slight case of diarrhea and frequently dragged her behind across the carpet. She was also scratching her ears quite often.

When I examined this little puppy, I immediately noticed her bloated stomach. She was much too skinny, and the skin around her eyes was drooping, a sure sign of poor health. A thick black crust covered the inside of her ears. This was clearly the result of tiny ear mites. I cleaned the inside of her ears with calendula oil and carefully massaged more oil into the base of the ears. I advised the owner to repeat this treatment every day at home. I sent a stool specimen to a laboratory to determine the type of parasites that were infesting the dog's intestinal system. The results showed a massive infestation of hookworms and spool worms. I gave the dog a powder made from several plants. The owner was to give this to the puppy for three days. We repeated this therapy three more times at ten-day intervals. In addition, I advised the owner to mix abrotanum 1× and garlic into Mona's food and to her own food that was easy to digest and high in calories for the next few days. Since worms remove large amounts of vitamin B from the body, for the next three days I gave the puppy injections of this life-sustaining vitamin, to which I added stimulants for the immune system.

One month later, Mona had gained 2lbs (1kg). A follow-up examination of her stool by the laboratory showed that she was free of all parasites. In addition, the insides of her ears were clear of ear mites.

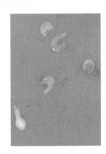

Above: These are single, excreted parts of tapeworms, but sometimes the parts are still attached to one another. When dry, they look almost like rice.

Below right: Dogs always attract ticks. Often, we don't detect them until they are quite large. The best way to remove them is to use a special pair of tweezers made just for this purpose.

Keeping Dogs Healthy

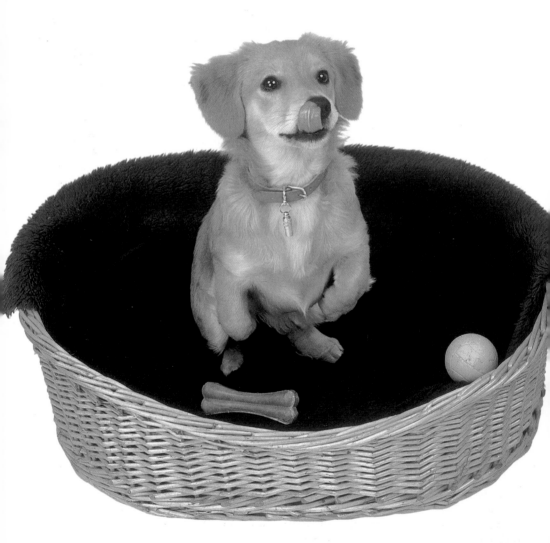

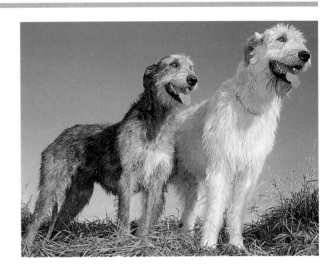

Dogs may be man's best friend, but that does not mean that they have forgotten that their ancestors were wolves. Their well-developed pack behavior has hardly changed after centuries of domestication. They are still extremely competitive.

Most dogs love to learn and do so quickly. Submissiveness, obedience to the head of the pack, and cooperation while hunting were important traits for survival within the original wolf pack. These traits are still evident in today's domesticated dog.

Each dog has its own characteristics. The person or family a dog lives with also influences these characteristics. The human family becomes the dog's "pack."

Although part of the development of a dog's character, or personality, depends on heredity, training and human contact are more influential. Innate viciousness is practically nonexistent. A dog will only overcome its instinct not to bite a human being after many bad experiences, after being mistreated, or if it has received systematic "attack training" from an irresponsible owner.

On the other hand, a responsible owner will raise a dog to be a friend by providing loving care and understanding, always keeping in mind the dog's inherited characteristics. Of course, the owner also is responsible for the health of his companion.

Male and Female Dogs

In addition to heredity and training, a dog's personality is strongly dependent on its gender. Sexual hormones are powerful influences controlling the way two dogs relate to each other. This is especially true of two dogs of the opposite sex. Until a dog's hormones have leveled off, which occurs at the end of puberty, we can't make accurate predictions about its temperament or love of adventure.

Purebred female dogs, such as this Irish wolfhound, are usually smaller and lighter than their male couterparts.

39

Two male dogs inspecting each other. The anal glands, located under the tail, produce the scents that act as a fragrant "calling card." A dog memorizes the scent of another dog, recognizing that scent years later.

TIP

A male dog that detects the scent of a female dog in heat loses all sense of obedience and runs after her. When you notice such a sudden outburst of sexual interest during a walk, hold on tight to the leash, and if necessary, grab your dog's collar.

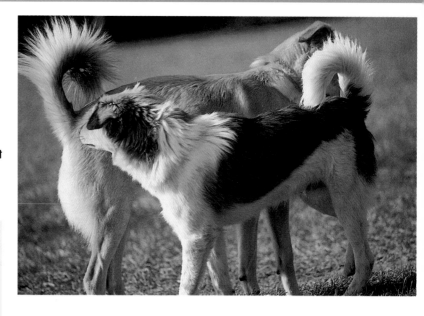

The Male Dog

Males and females of the same breed differ in body size and stature. A male dog is usually larger, heavier, and more compact. However, that only holds true for purebreds; mixed breeds are another matter.

In general, male dogs are fully developed sexually by the time they are eight to twelve months old. During puberty, their behavior is not all that different from their human counterparts, always wanting to impress their comrades. (See "Developmental Stages of a Young Dog," pages 28 and 29.)

Interest in female dogs increaes steadily during this time. Once the sexual drive is fully devleoped, nothing can separate a male from a female dog in heat. When he smells the urine left behind by a female dog in heat, he will lift his head and stare far into the distance. His teeth may chatter, and saliva may drip from his mouth. No fence is too high, and no river is too wide for him. Unless he is on a leash, he will run blindly, sometimes for hundreds of miles, after the female that left such an attractive fragrance behind.

Adult male dogs usually view each other as rivals. When they meet, they try to impress each other with their raised fur, bared teeth, and ferocious growls.

Often dogs progress from trying to impress each other to real fighting. Although serious injuries are rare, don't take the danger of infection from bites lightly. We discuss the treatment of such injuries in detail in "Case Histories," page 59.

In general, male dogs need more consistent and stronger discipline, and they take longer than female dogs to learn the basics (housebreaking, walking on a leash, and showing submission to the owner) and to obey commands reliably. Furthermore, male dogs need a stronger "hand" so that they don't misunderstand their relationship with the people in their family.

Among other things, the male hormone, testosterone, determines how aggressive a male dog will be. For that reason, neutering usually produces a much gentler male dog. The surgical removal of the testicles, however, may diminish a dog's sense of adventure and his energy level. Neutered dogs, therefore, should not be fed as much food as those that have not been castrated. This surgery, performed at the veterinarian's office, is a routine procedure.

The Female Dog

Purebred female dogs are usually smaller and lighter in weight than their male counterparts. With mixed breeds, weight and size are difficult to predict. During puberty, female dogs, too, can misbehave and sometimes even be rebellious. A very self-confident female dog

False Pregnancy

Even if the female did not conceive during copulation, she may show signs as if she were pregnant. A false pregnancy may cause a female dog to show her owner greater affection but be more aggressive towards strangers than normal. If the behavior is disturbing, you may need to obtain medication from your veterinarian or practitioner. Milk secretion from the nipples also occurs in false pregnancies. You'll find a discussion of the help available for that problem available in "Case Histories," page 54.

will constantly try to act as if she were the head of the "pack." You'll have to be unrelenting and consistent in order to train her to remember that you are the boss. In general, disobedience and opposition to people during this time are not as strong as in males of the same age.

The behavior of the female dog to another differs from one animal to the next. Many female dogs remain friendly or at least do not become aggressive towards other adult female dogs. When they are not in heat, they behave the same way towards male dogs. However, some females turn into real roughnecks and will start trouble with every dog that comes along.

Above: Here a male dog sniffs the anal region of a female dog. Whether a female allows this depends on their respective ranks. Male dogs that are higher in rank may sniff female dogs that are lower in rank.

Below: If a female dog is not in heat, she refuses the anal test by simply sitting down.

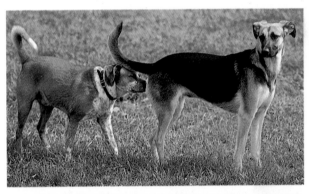

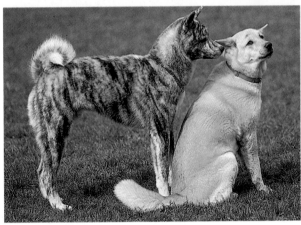

41

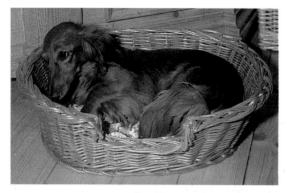 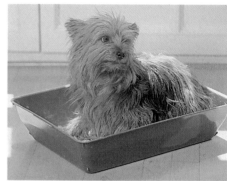

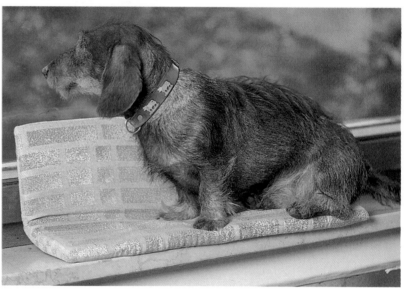

Above left: Every dog needs a place with a blanket to call its own.

Above right: A small dog can easily use a cat litter box now and then, but this should never replace a daily walk outside.

Below: A seat on the windowsill with a view is entertaining, offering some diversion to a dog left alone.

For most female dogs, the first sign of heat appears when they are six to eight months old. With most breeds, the female is fully developed at ten to twelve months. From then on, they come into heat twice every year. In some cases, especially with the larger breeds, the interval between each heat cycle might be every eight to ten months. The intensity of the physical signs also differs from one dog to another. The vaginal opening becomes enlarged and a clear discharge appears. This becomes bloody later. To humans, the discharge is odorless. Male dogs show a great deal of interest in this discharge because it signals that the female is almost ready for copulation.

At this point in the cycle, the female dog is not at all receptive to the overtures of a male dog. She will not be ready to mate and conceive until nine to thirteen days after she starts to bleed.

If you want to avoid a parade of male dogs at your door whenever your female

Neutering

Castration, usually thought of in relation to males, simply means that the surgeon removes the gonads. In a female animal that means the removal of the ovaries and frequently the uterus; in a male animal, the surgeon removes the testicles. Since the gonads produce the sexual hormones, this form of neutering prevents reproduction, and the absence of the hormones removes the sexual drive. Spaying similarly refers to a surgical procedure for both males and females: the surgeon only ties the female's fallopian tubes or the male's vas deferens. While spaying will definitely prevent conception, it doesn't affect the heat cycle of the female or the turbulent behavior of the male. In that sense, spaying is of little help. The owner of a female dog in heat must still keep the dog on a leash or lock her away, or she will take off with her "beloved," disappearing over the hills.

The owner of a male dog must still track his pet to the front door of the female in heat, joining the ranks of all the other owners of neighborhood male dogs.

Another method of preventing unintended pregnancies involves hormone treatments. The veterinarian may give the female dog a tablet or an injection. However, when used over a prolonged period of time, this method may produce severe side effects.

TIP

Always keep a leash on a female dog in heat when you take her out for a walk, because even the most obedient and faithful female will take off with a potential mate.

dog is in heat, try carrying her several blocks away from the house and walking her there. Of course, you'll have to reverse the procedure when you bring her home. This will interrupt the trail of her scent, denying male dogs her home address. If you want to avoid the recurring stress of keeping male dogs off your front lawn and save your female dog the frustration of an unsatisfied sexual drive, you might want to have her neutered. As in the case for neutered male dogs, neutered females require fewer calories. On the other hand, if you want to breed your female dog, wait until she is at least eighteen months old, when her physical development is complete. In theory, a female dog is able to have puppies until she is quite old; however, complications are more frequent for dog mothers over the age of six years. These complications occur both during the pregnancy and at birth.

Keeping a Dog Inside

Sharing your house or apartment with a dog is not a problem because of the variety of shapes and sizes of both purebreds and mixed breeds. However, a dog that spends most of its time inside needs more attention. The owner must take it for extended walks and provide enough playtime. Otherwise, the dog becomes bored in an environment that is rather

TIP

Joining a dog club may help you deal with a dog showing signs of disturbed behavior.

Just like people, dogs can have psychological problems that result in unusual or unacceptable behavior. In general the cause of the problem has more to do with the dog's immediate environment, lifestyle, and with mistakes made by the people who take care of the dog than it does with the dog's character or personality. Traumatic experiences that occurred when the dog was young can leave a permanent impression on the psyche and cause behavioral problems, particularly if such experiences continue.

Here are the most frequent problems:

Aggressiveness Towards People

In a very few cases, organic brain damage is the reason for aggressive behavior towards people. Usually, the mistakes made while training the young dog or puppy are the cause. An aggressive dog thinks that it is the leader of the pack and that its growling and biting puts the lower-ranked humans in their place. People often think a small dog is cute if it defends its food and toys with fierce growls. But when, as often happens, the same dog bites the owner, people think the dog is vicious.

While Bach flower remedies might be useful for support, you can only achieve real change with consistent, if belated, training. You must use the proper discipline to teach the dog

Behavioral

that it is the lowest-ranked member in the "pack" and that is must subordinate itself to the people in the family.

Fear-based Biting

While fear-based biting is as dangerous to people, especially to children, as it is to other dogs, the reason for this behavioral problem lies somewhere else. Although such behavior might be an inherited character flaw, most often it is due to bad experiences the dog had as a puppy or young adult. In the majority of cases, repeated frightening experiences, extreme physical stress, or abuse is the cause.

You'll have to teach the dog not to react to every insignificant event as if its life were in danger. The dog must learn not to panic and attack whoever if feels is threatening it. Attacks help the dog develop a sense of self-confidence. But changing the behavior requires a considerable amount of sensitivity so that the dog does not think that it can move up in rank in the family "pack." Games which allow the dog to be the winner, such as retrieval exercises, are a good way to increase its self-confidence. Letting a male dog play with females that are peaceful does much to bolster a male's own image. If a dog always bites when faced with a particular situation, try to simulate that situation as often as possible in a playful way. Lavish praise and rewards will encourage better behavior.

Housebreaking Problems

your dog urinates and defecates in the house, you must first eliminate any possible physical problems. Aging dogs often suffer from incontinence. However, kidney and bladder diseases and heart problems are the main causes of "accidents."

The most common psychological reason for a dog to have trouble with housebreaking is fear. When an adult dog continuously relieves itself indoors because of fear, it is very likely that someone severely and repeatedly mistreated the dog in the past. Such a dog needs an enormous amount of love, patience, and attention. Punishing the dog is the worst thing you can do. It doesn't work and actually make matters worse. The only remedy is to strengthen the dog's trust and self-confidence with lots of praise and reassurance or to let it play with smaller, nonaggressive dogs.

Excessive Aggression Towards Other Dogs

Unfortunately, some dogs are notorious roughnecks. Such dogs are usually self-confident, dominant males that will attack any other males that cross their path. But some female dogs are also aggressive towards other dogs. Some breeds, such as boxers, dachshunds, Akitas, and Doberman pinschers, are somewhat more disposed toward such bad habits. When such an aggressive dog also inherits a character weakness or lacks obedience, seemingly harmless roughhousing may quickly turn into a very serious and bloody fight. This type of dog needs to be on a leash (and perhaps even muzzled) whenever it is outside, to protect the owner and the rest of the neighborhood dog population.

Even a puppy needs to have contact with many other dogs, because contact, play, and experiences with members of its own species are vital for the psychological health of an animal. This is especially important for miniature breeds, because, if you pick up a small dog every time a larger dog comes along, the dog will develop a misguided sense of strength and size. The inevitable result is a constantly yapping small dog that is an embarrassment to its owner. What is worse, the dog is in danger because it thinks it can defeat every other dog, no matter what the size.

Owners who work outside the house have a particular problem. Dogs are social animals by nature, and they will literally become lonely if they are left alone for more than four or five hours. The result is often constant barking or whining, destruction of furniture, or "accidents" in the house. Only very self-confident and well-trained dogs are able to be alone for long periods of time without sustaining psychological damage. The least that the owner owes a dog that is alone for more than five hours is lots of praise and as much play as possible.

TIP

Chasing bicycles or other vehicles is a bad habit resulting from a frustrated hunting instinct. Giving the dog more opportunities to play (for example, retrieving or shaking a bag) helps the dog use this instinct in a harmless way.

45

TIP

Nutrition

In general, dogs thrive on commercial dog food. This food contains everything your dog needs to be healthy, provided that you give the amount recommended by the manufacturer.

Important: Canned food contains chemical additives. Do not give canned food to dogs that have allergies. Dogs with kidney and bladder problems, on the other hand, should not eat dry food since they will have to drink more water.

If you want to provide home-cooked food for your adult dog, you must make sure that you satisfy its nutritional requirements. A dog's food must contain meat, vegetables, grains, minerals, vitamins, and trace elements.

You need to provide the basic nutritional substances in the following ratio: carbohydrates—fifty percent; protein—thirty percent; fat—five percent; fiber—five percent; and calcium and phosphate—two percent.

Important: Do not feed your dog raw meat, because raw meat can cause food poisoning from salmonella or viral infections.

The amount of food your dog needs depends, of course, on its size, weight, and life-style. Ask your veterinarian or practitioner for advice. As a general rule, adult dogs should maintain their ideal weight, not losing or gaining any weight. A dog's last two ribs ought to be visible through its skin.

Normal Weight (in pounds)	Caloric Intake
4.5 (2 kg)	240
11 (5 kg)	450
22 (10 kg)	750
66 (30 kg)	1710

monotonous compared to the outside world. The more space a dog has for running, sniffing, playing around, and being with other dogs, the better off both of you will be.

The Outdoor Dog

Keeping your dog outside in a kennel is perfectly acceptable. As a matter of fact, a few breeds, such as Newfoundland dogs and Saint Bernards, are actually more comfortable if they are kept outside. However, if you keep your dog outside permanently, you must make sure that the dog does not lose its contact with the "family pack." Only daily contact with the animal, including daily playtime and regular walks, keeps the dog psychologically healthy. To own a dog simply to protect your house without allowing the dog to have a close relationship with the family borders on cruelty.

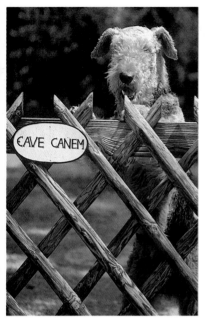

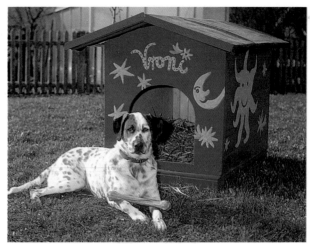

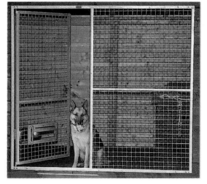

If you want to keep your dog outside, you need to pay attention to the following:

- Your dog must have fresh drinking water available at all times.
- In addition to a doghouse, your dog needs a dry and shady place where it can rest.
- You must remove leftover food and excrement daily.
- You need to have the dog and its sleeping quarters examined for parasites at regular, frequent intervals.
- You need to inspect the kennel, the leash or chain, and any fence regularly to avoid possible injuries.

These are the very basic, minimum requirements necessary for the health of a dog that lives outside on a permanent basis. But true loving care also includes regular walks, plenty of attention, toys, and good nutrition.

Of course, sick and very old dogs do not belong outside in a kennel or on a chain. In general, female dogs in the last third of their pregnancy and nursing dogs should not be tied up outside. Dogs should not be kept outside on a chain or in any area without a roof during periods of prolonged rain.

The Doghouse

Whether you keep your dog on a chain, in a kennel, or let it roam freely in the backyard, it always needs a doghouse for

Left: Many dogs that live outside are responsible for protecting the house and property.

Above right: Dogs that are kept outside, whether permanently or some of the time, need a doghouse. Some doghouses are real eye-catchers.

Below right: At least one side of a kennel must face the yard in order for the dog to have an unobstructed view of its surroundings.

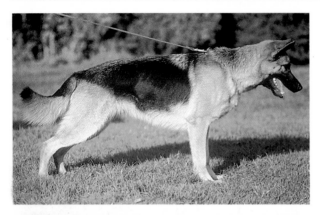

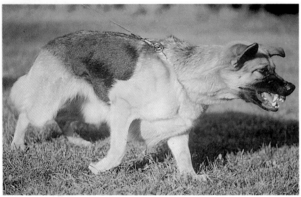

Parasites

Dogs, just like all other animals, are bothered by numerous parasites. External parasites—like fleas and mites—are found in or on the surface of the skin. Internal parasites—worms and microscopically small single-cell organisms—can infest the intestines or other internal organs. What they all have in common is that they are all capable of weakening the host, often causing many different illnesses and much suffering.

For that reason, it is absolutely essential that the owner adhere to a regular deworming schedule. (See also "Immunization and Deworming," page 24.) If the animal sleeps on a pillow or pads, make sure to replace them regularly; they are a favorite nesting place for parasites. A dog blanket should be washable. In addition, early detection is easier when fur and skin are checked during routine care. (See also "Prevention," page 76.)

Above: An alert and aggressive dog is protecting an object.

Below: Even someone who knows little about dog behavior would know that this dog is ready to attack.

shelter. The doghouse needs to be big enough so that the dog can comfortably turn around in it, but it must also be small enough that even in the dead of winter its own body heat will keep it warm. The outside walls, the floor, and the roof ought to be watertight and insulated. During the winter months, you should provide a layer of straw or an insulating pad (available in pet stores) for added comfort. Attaching a blanket to the top of the entrance to the doghouse and brushes to the sides will also be helpful. The brushes will remove snow from the dog's coat when it enters the doghouse, keeping the inside dry.

The building materials should not contain toxic substances and should not splinter, because many dogs will chew on the wood when they are bored. Be sure that no nails or screws protrude.

The best place for a doghouse is in an area that has shade and is protected from the wind. Place the doghouse so that your dog has a good view of the surroundings that it is supposed to protect. If possible, the doghouse entrance should face south or at least away from the side exposed to bad weather. The ground underneath and around the doghouse should not collect water when it rains. A gravel or a cement floor is best. You can safely raise the doghouse off the ground by placing bricks under each of the corners.

Keeping Your Dog in the Backyard

Make sure that your dog won't be hurt by a fence or by tools left on the ground. A fence needs to be high enough so that neither your dog nor a strange dog can jump over it. It must also be strong enough so that the dog can't break it or squeeze through it. Two dogs can seriously injure each other even with a fence between them. Fences made from wooden slats work well, provided that the slats are close enough together.

Dogs on a Chain or in a Kennel

You should not chain your dog every day. Being on a chain is very unnatural because it severely hinders the animal's movements. The only exception should be if the dog poses a danger to people, to other animals, or if the dog itself is in danger.

If you intend to tie up your dog, be sure to follow the previous instructions. Keeping your dog in a kennel for long periods of time is a problem. A dog in a kennel has less freedom of movement and less opportunity for diversion than it would if it were only chained up. However, using a kennel once in a while is perfectly acceptable, as long as the kennel is clean, the kennel staff take the dog

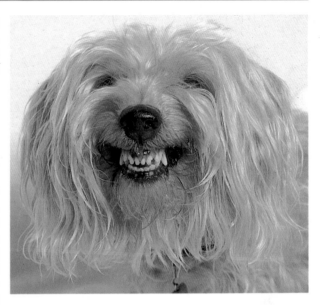

for walks, and the handlers maintain contact with the dog. A dog weighing 45lbs (20kg) needs a kennel of at least 65sq ft (6sq m), and the width must be at least the same as the dog's length.

Dog Language

To be responsible dog owners, the members of a "family pack" have to understand their dog's "language." Here is a discussion of a few important "words" in a dog's language:

A dog's bark sounds different in different situations. The bark may be an invitation to come and play, a greeting, or a warning. The meaning of a growl is more obvious. It can be a warning that the dog will attack, or it can mean that there is danger ahead. The combination of bared

Whether or not a dog is about to attack is not always obvious with dogs that have long, floppy ears or long hair. This one is baring its teeth, ready to bite.

TIP

Since different breeds have very different appearances, including the length of the coat and the shape of the head and ears, you need to spend some time observing a dog to understand its "language."

Above: When the owner consistently uses hand signals to emphasize a command, the dog has an easier time learning.

Below: Good training helps prevent traffic accidents. A dog should learn to "sit" at every curb before crossing the street.

TIP

Take precaution when walking near the woods: The scent of wild animals sometimes makes even the best-trained dog forget his training. Keep him leashed.

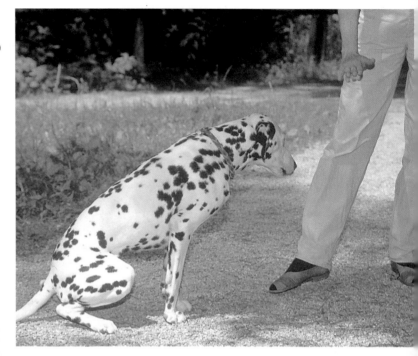

teeth, raised fur, and growling indicates that the dog is very excited. Yelping and whining mean that it is in pain, physically or psychologically. If, however, the dog yelps or whines when something positive is happening, it wants attention, and it wants to be petted.

Generally, a dog expresses fear by flattening its ears and tucking its tail between its legs. In addition, the dog may crouch, making itself smaller. Be careful, because a dog that is afraid may also bite.

A self-confident dog makes itself big, stands very straight, and stretches slightly forward. An aggressive dog holds its tail vertically, stretches its head forward, and raises its fur. A dog that is ready to attack (and one that is not afraid) holds its tail straight up, points its ears forward slightly, and bares its teeth.

When a dog sits down, it is either evaluating the situation or has lost inter-

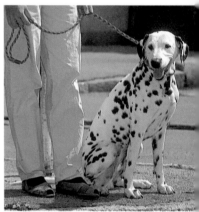

est. When a dog lies down and shows its unprotected belly, it is signaling sub missiveness towards the opponent, saying, "Don't attack me, I surrender." Often when a dog shows its belly to a person the dog is saying, "Please rub my tummy."

And last, but not least, when a dog wags its tail and seems to almost curtsy in front of you, it is saying, "It's time to play"—an activity important for body and soul.

Dog Training

A very important part of owning a dog is proper training. That should start when the dog is still very young. The reasons for starting young and some of the basic rules are discussed in "Fourth to Sixth Month," page 27.

Training should always be fun, and rewards should play a major role. The result will be a dog that will obey eagerly and will view its owner as the "master," rather then simply following commands out of fear. Constant pressure, force, and punishment destroy a dog psychologically.

A basic goal of training should be to teach the dog to "stay behind," meaning to be alone for four to five hours at a time. Longer than that could result in behavioral problems.

Learning to walk on a leash and to "sit" are particularly important for a city dog. Before you allow your dog to walk without a leash, it should know the commands "Sit" and "Come," meaning that it must come to you when told to do so.

TIP

You can teach a dog not to pull on the leash by yanking it back with a short and powerful tug. If your dog is big and strong, don't be too timid when doing this.

Your dog won't be able to connect the punishment with the deed unless you catch the dog in the act, as here, stealing a box of cookies.

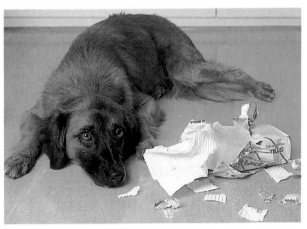

TIP

You'll find more detailed information about the use of therapeutic methods (compresses, inhalation, etc.) and about nursing care (such as taking temperature) in "Nursing Care," pages 78 to 95.

The Most Frequently

Recognizable Symptoms	Possible Reasons
Yellow or watery secretion from eyes, combined with severe sensitivity; highly inflamed or extremely pale conjunctiva	Conjunctivitis caused by bacterial infection, foreign object embedded in the eye, allergies, injury to the cornea; heart trouble or chronic disease of internal organs; parasite invasion
Yellow, possibly bloody discharge from the nose; frequent sneezing	Foreign object embedded in the nose; allergies; tumor
Black, sticky layer inside the ears; foul odor; constantly shaking the head (itching)	Ear mite infection; infection of ear canal (particularly in dog with floppy, long ears); bloody ear
Frequently scratching, licking, biting the fur; black or white objects attached to the fur; bare spots with or without scabs; frequent and incessant scratching (itching)	Skin parasites such as lice, fleas, or skin mites; skin fungus or allergies; hormone imbalance; psychological problems
Swelling under the skin	Abscess; tumor; cyst (swelling under the skin due to accumulation of fat in the tissues)
Refuses to eat and displays obvious quiet behavior; restlessness, frequent whining; refuses to lie down; turning around on the stomach (specifically in large breeds)	Beginning of a general illness, or one involving internal organs; in female dogs, pseudopregnancy or infection of the uterus
Rapid weight loss; alternating between ravenous hunger and loss of appetite; bloated belly, noisy sounds in the stomach and intestines	Pancreas disease; parasite invasion of the intestinal tract; flatulence
Discharge in the genital area; frequent urge to urinate without producing urine	Female dogs, uterus infection; male dogs, prostate problems; kidney and bladder infection
Dog drags hindquarters over the ground; anus covered with sticky crusted material; slightly opened sphincter muscle; no tail motion	Clogged or inflamed rectal lymph nodes; parasite infection of the intestinal tract; slight paralysis caused by spinal injury
Lame leg or paw; difficulty lifting leg and/or lying or sitting down	Sprained, bruised, or torn tendon; lameness due to nerve injury; arthritis
Diarrhea	Spoiled food, poison, or eating too much snow; liver or pancreas problems; food allergies
Vomiting	Spoiled food, poison, or eating too much snow; ingested foreign object; food allergies; problems in the internal organs

Occurring Illnesses

What You Can Do	See Your Veterinarian If
Cool compresses with chamomile tea; give *Euphrasia* several times a day	You can't rule out possible injury or ingestion of a foreign object; no improvement in the next three days; symptoms worsen
Let the dog inhale steam from chamomile tea; give Traumeel pills several times a day; take temperature	Always, for proper diagnosis
Apply oxygenated olive oil or calendula oil to the nose several times a day, massaging it into the base of the ear	No improvement within three days; symptoms worsen; accompanied by severe swelling or pain
In the presence of parasites: treat with commercial flea powder; feed plenty of garlic	No evidence of parasites; no improvement within three days; severe skin infection
In the presence of an abscess, give *Hepar sulfuris* 8 × to bring it to a head; to heal, *Hepar sulfuris* 12 × or *Myristica sebifera* 63 × several times a day	Always, to determine if it is an abscess or a tumor
Take temperature; watch the dog closely; if ingested foreign object or in case of stomach problems, withhold food; treat with medication that strengthens the immune system, such as *Echinacea*	Situation is unclear; foreign object ingested; in cases of stomach problems; no improvement within two hours; symptoms recur; temperature above 103°F (39.5°C) or below 100.5°F (38°C)
Take temperature; deworm regularly; in case of flatulence, add caraway seeds, fennel, and anise to food	Other symptoms appear; flatulence appears frequently; you suspect worm infestation; temperature above 103°F (39.5°C) or below 100.5°F (38°C)
Take temperature; give *Echinacea*; in case of bladder problems, give Indian kidney tea	Always, to establish a proper diagnosis and to initiate effective treatment
In case of rectal lymph node problems, apply cool, wet compresses with anise or chamomile tea; use a regular deworming schedule	No improvement within two days; symptoms worsen
Cold compresses with arnica tincture; give Traumeel tablets every two hours until dog improves, then give only several times a day; in case of injury to a nerve: give *Hypericum* 0 × or 2 ×	Bone fractured or ligaments or nerve injured; still lame after three days or if lameness recurs; bites; wounds are large, deep, and wide
Take temperature; for twenty-four hours, give only chamomile or black tea, then for few days, feed a light diet (fish, chicken, rice); watch the dog carefully; give immune-stimulating medication, such as *Echinacea* or Kaopectate, several times a day	No actual improvements within two days; other symptoms appear; you cannot rule out poisoning; temperature above 103°F (39.5°C) or below 100.5°F (38°C)
Take temperature; for twenty-four hours, give only peppermint tea, then feed a light diet (fish, chicken, rice); watch the animal carefully; several times a day give *Nux vomica D6* and/or *Echinacea*	No actual improvements within two days; other symptoms appear; you cannot rule out poisoning or ingestion of foreign object; temperature above 103°F (39.5°C) or below 100.5°F (38°C)

TIP

You'll find more detailed information about natural remedies in "Natural Healing Remedies in Your Medicine Cabinet," pages 16 and 17.

Case Histories from My Practice

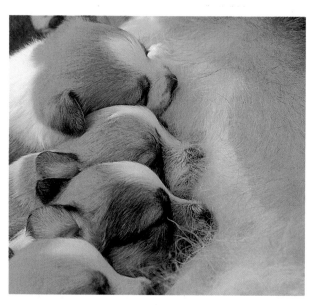

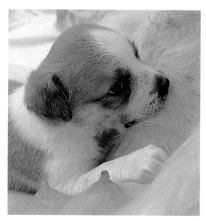

Left: Sometimes puppies injure their mother's nipples.

Right: Healthy nipples are soft, allowing the puppies to extract milk without overexertion.

Inflammation of the Nipples

A nursing mother's infected nipples are not only painful for her but also dangerous for the puppies, because, in general, the mother's milk carries the germs responsible for the infection. In addition, puppies have a difficult time getting milk out of the hardened nipples. Sometimes, they can't get any milk out at all. If we detect this type of infection and its complications too late, the puppies may starve to death, or they may suck so hard that the nipples are literally eaten away.

Not long ago, the owner of a four-year-old female dog asked me to come to her house. The dog, Bella, had just given birth to a litter of puppies. I went immediately because she thought something was wrong with the dog's nipples. When I examined Bella, I discovered that the nipples on the right side were hot and swollen. I was only able to squeeze a few drops of milk from them. In addition, the dog had a slightly elevated temperature. Although her puppies were restless, they showed no signs yet of being dehydrated. While I applied cold, wet com-

54

presses to the inflamed nipples, I told the owner how she could best supplement the food for the puppies. I also gave the whole family injections of a plant extract to increase their own defense mechanisms. In addition, the owner was to give the mother dog a special homeopathic medication every two hours and to reduce that to three times a day after the symptoms showed improvement. The owner was also to apply arnica compresses three times a day.

The next day the nipples were considerably softer. In spite of the improvement, I repeated the immune-stimulating injections on the second day. After two more days, all symptoms of the inflammation of the nipples had disappeared, and the puppies did not need any more supplemental feedings.

mites on to another dog (but not to humans), these parasites tend to attack sick dogs and those with weak immune systems more frequently than healthy animals.

Leslie, an eighteen-month-old mixed breed, had come home two months ago from vacation with her owner. She looked rather poorly and neglected when she arrived home. She had been dewormed and immunized previously, but she still had hair-root mites. The owner wanted me to rid the dog of these pests once and for all.

I could clearly see large, bare, crusty patches above her eyes and mouth. During my examination, I found two more infected areas between the toes. I found no symptoms of other problems, other than the infestation.

Incessant licking often indicates that the dog itches. This behavior usually indicates the presence of external parasites or allergies. However, dogs may also develop a licking habit that is rooted in psychological problems.

Hair-root Mite Infestation

The hair-root mite, scientific name *Demodex*, is one of the three types of mites that infest dogs. This is a skin mite that bores into the uppermost layer of the skin, where it lives and creates virtual tunnels. Wherever it appears, it causes inflammation and loss of hair. The mite is so small you cannot detect it with the naked eye. You need to examine the skin under a microscope to make a diagnosis.

Hair-root mites are particularly difficult to treat because they are resistant to many of the available medications. Unfortunately, treatment takes a long time and requires patience and a consistent effort. While one dog can easily pass the

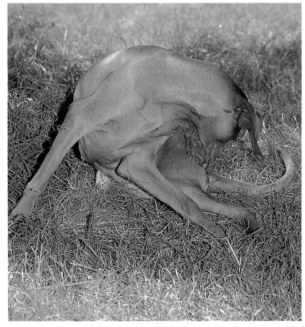

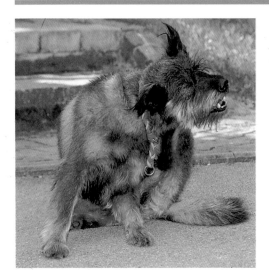
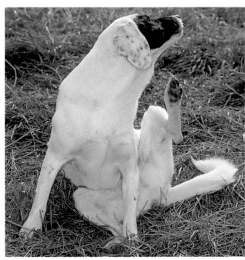

Left: Ear mites are usually the reason a dog shakes its head severely and frequently.

Right: A dog that scratches itself frequently and severely is trying to get rid of a bad itch. The animal often injures the skin, leading to an inflammation or an infection.

I treated the mite-infected dog with a "soft laser" and decided on a program of acupuncture once a week. I applied oxygenated olive oil to the affected skin areas and instructed the owner to continue applying the oil every day. In order to improve the dog's overall physical condition and to strengthen Leslie's own defense mechanism, I gave her an injection once a week which consisted of a plant-based immune-stimulating medication, enzymes, and homeopathic remedies. In addition, I suggested that the owner add garlic extract and a vitamin B supplement to the dog's food.

Within three weeks, we noticed a considerable improvement in the affected area of the skin. Leslie had gained weight, and her fur was shiny. Three weeks later, all the hair had grown back on her face, and Leslie turned into an absolutely beautiful young dog. The only place where the mite infection remained was between two toes and in the nail bed of one of those toes. For that reason, we continued treatment as before. The para-

sites proved to be especially obstinate in that area. Two more months passed before all the symptoms disappeared.

Flea Allergies

Dogs often play host to fleas, and some dogs have allergic reactions to flea bites. The bites can cause inflammations or even widespread eczema. The intense itching caused by flea bites causes equally intense scratching or biting of the affected area. The scratching or biting gives rise to inflammation. The itching increases because of the incessant scratching, and the dog will scratch even more. Obviously, this becomes a vicious cycle. Untreated, these inflammations may turn into very nasty infections that affect the whole organism.

Chronic Ear Infections

Chronic ear infections are more common in dogs with long ears, such as basset hounds and cocker spaniels, than in dogs with shorter ears. Long, floppy ears prevent sufficient air from reaching the ear canal, creating a moist and warm environment that, combined with natural ear wax, is an ideal place for bacteria to thrive. An ear infection is usually accompanied by a foul odor. Yellow pus and sensitivity to pressure at the base of the ears are additional signs of an ear infection.

You can treat such infections with natural remedies. In advanced cases, however, the dog may need surgery.

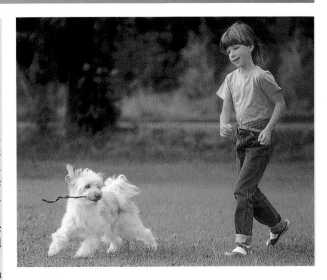

Fortunately, James, a male Irish setter, brought to my office by his very concerned owner, had not yet reached such a state. For two weeks the owner had treated him with commercial flea powder. The treatment had not worked. The dog continued to scratch himself furiously, and both fleas and their droppings were still visible in his fur.

When I examined him, I found several flea bites on his belly. In some areas, the skin was inflamed, and wet secretions were also visible. The fur on both sides of his body had already lost some of its color because of the constant presence of saliva, and the fur was almost totally gone on the inside hind legs and the back of the knees. I found scabs in several places on the skin. Nevertheless, the dog seemed to be rather healthy. In order to lessen the itching, I decided to use acupuncture once a week. Every third day, I gave the dog injections consisting of a combination of vitamin B and ophidian extract. I asked the owner to bathe the dog with shampoo made from different plant extracts (thyme and rosemary) that are effective against flea infestation and healing earth that would soothe the inflamed skin. In addition, I asked him to carefully comb the dog's fur with a flea comb, give him an organ-enzyme medication daily, and add garlic tablets and plenty of vitamin A to his food.

In only a few weeks, the owner noticed that James was scratching himself much less and that the condition of the skin was much improved. After five injections, all symptoms had disappeared. To make sure that the dog was rid of all fleas, the owner bathed him with the above-mentioned shampoo. Since a tapeworm can serve as an interim host for fleas, the owner had James dewormed four weeks later and then again eight weeks after that.

Because broken branches can easily injure a dog's mouth, use more substantial objects for retrieving.

Above: Chicken bones, which your dog may think of as a delicacy, can be extremely dangerous because they splinter when chewed. The splinters can cause very dangerous injuries.

Below: Rank plays a very important role among canines. Fights are one means of establishing rank. If dogs have learned how to behave around each other, such fights are usually not bloody.

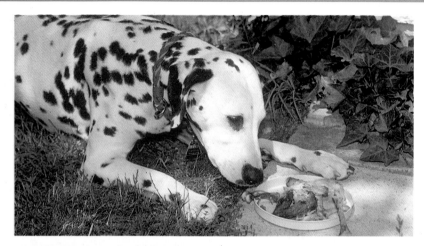

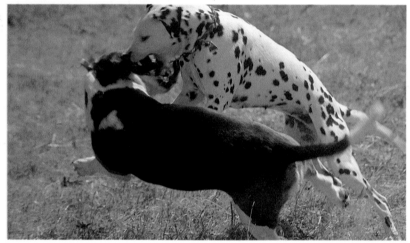

Ingested Foreign Objects

Dogs frequently swallow foreign objects while chewing on them or while playing with them. In most cases, these objects are part of larger bones or pieces of balls and other toys. With any luck, a swallowed object will pass through the digestive system, and the dog will excrete it naturally. However, all too often, a swallowed object obstructs the stomach or the digestive system or even breaks through an intestinal wall. When this is the case, unless the object is removed by surgery or with an endoscope, the dog will have an intestinal blockage or peritonitis. Both of these complications are almost always fatal.

The owner of Charlie, a two-year-old Saint Bernard, reported that his dog had been chewing on a hard rubber ball and had swallowed some of the pieces. Later, he vomited several times. I immediately took X rays. These showed several small pieces of rubber at the base of the stomach with a larger piece lodged in the intestines. Since the dog was still lively and well, didn't show any sign of pain in the stomach, and was still passing stool, surgery was not immediately necessary. Instead, I tried to help the dog pass the rubber pieces the natural way. I gave Charlie a large amount of whipped potatoes and cotton balls. To counteract the nausea that was sure to follow, I gave the dog an injection of a homeopathic medication and requested that the owner give him the same medication in suppository form at home.

I asked the owner to contact me immediately if the dog's condition worsened. The following evening, Charlie did indeed take a turn for the worse. I alerted a veterinarian friend of mine, who operated immediately. To strengthen the dog's immune system, I gave him an injection of a plant extract as well as arnica 4 × to limit the amount of blood loss during surgery and to support wound healing. We gave the dog the same medication over the next two days. To minimize the shock of the operation, I also prescribed Bach Flower Rescue Remedy. To lessen the pain, I gave Charlie a combination of a plant remedies. Ten days after surgery, the wound had healed beautifully, and I removed the sutures. In no time at all, Charlie was running and playing, as lively as ever; only now, playing with a rubber ball was out—for good!

Bites

Since dogs, particularly male dogs, have an instinctive need to establish who is

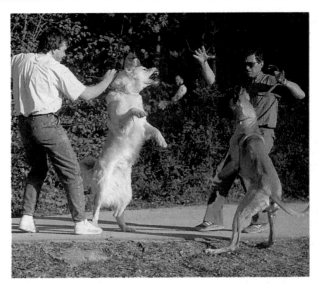

the boss, they often test their courage and power in furiously fought battles. Such fights, however, are still subject to the laws established long ago by their common ancestor, the wolf, and serious or even fatal injuries seldom occur, provided that the animals still possess their instincts. However, deep bites are not uncommon in these confrontations. Because of the danger of infection, we must treat such injuries.

The owner of Tibor, a male rottweiler, was right to bring the dog to my office. Tibor had been part of a real street fight. Tibor was a very domineering dog. Threatening postures by other dogs never impressed him; he always was ready for a fight. This particular time, however, he had met his match. In the ensuing fight, both dogs received injuries.

When I examined Tibor's body for bleeding wounds, I found the impression of his opponent's teeth on Tibor's neck and shoulder. Luckily, only two teeth had penetrated deep into the muscles; the

A dog on a leash usually feels much more courageous than one that is running free. In addition, two leashed dogs cannot approach each other the way they normally would. Thus, they do not often get into serious fights.

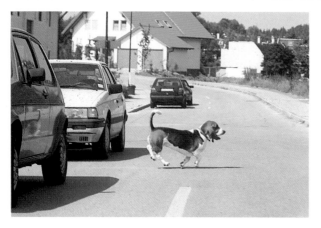

Cars are the most common cause of injuries to dogs. Training your dog properly is the best prevention.

the latter in tablet form several times a day. In addition, I advised him to keep an eye on the deeper wounds and to make sure that they didn't start to develop a surface scab prematurely, which would lead to an abscess.

We repeated this treatment protocol on the second day. The superficial wounds had already begun to heal, and the deeper wounds remained free of infection. His owner brought Tibor to my office every two or three days for observation. Ten days later, all the wounds had healed completely.

rest had only scratched the skin. He also had small, superficial wounds on his head. I cleaned the more serious injuries with a diluted iodine solution and thoroughly disinfected all the wounds. Then I gave the dog an injection of a plant extract to strengthen his immune system. I also used a homeopathic remedy to support the healing process and lessen the pain. I asked the owner to give Tibor

Behavioral Problems

A dog's physical problems are seldom the cause for its behavioral problems.

Traffic Accidents

Traffic accidents are the most common cause of injuries to dogs. Females in heat and love-stricken males are particularly vulnerable because, when the time comes for mating, they are unable to obey any command. However, a poorly trained dog that won't listen is much more likely to run into the street and be hit by a car.

Fortunately, modern surgical methods can save the lives of many dogs and can prevent serious disabilities. For that reason, I usually refer animals injured in accidents to a veterinarian or an animal clinic, but not before I treat the animal for shock. An animal that goes into shock as a result of an accident doesn't get all of the oxygen it needs for survival. Often Bach Flower Rescue Remedy is helpful in dealing with such a situation.

Health practitioners also use plant extract as well as electrolyte infusion to support the heart and circulatory system. We use ophidian extract and arnica 4 × to help stop bleeding, particularly internal bleeding.

The most effective care a practitioner can provide, however, is postoperative treatment with natural remedies.

Most behavioral problems result from traumatic experiences that occurred when the dog was a puppy, including improper handling, abuse, or a change in the "family pack."

Several of these factors had influenced Roy, a fifteen-month-old male German shepherd. About three months before, the owner had found Roy in an animal shelter. The records indicated that the previous owner had repeatedly abused the dog physically. Roy accepted his new home immediately and was very obedient towards the new owner. However, he wouldn't go near her husband and refused to follow his commands. During the course of a family dispute, the dog became aggressive towards the husband.

I helped them understand that Roy had obviously accepted the wife as the "boss of the pack," but he considered the husband to be at the bottom of the rank. Ray may have felt this way because the woman had picked him up at the animal shelter while her husband was away, and the husband hadn't met him until two days later. For the sake of safety and of a peaceful house, the young male dog needed to learn that he was the lowest member of the pack and that he needed to obey both wife and husband.

I suggested that only the husband should feed the dog and take him for his daily walks for several days. The more the husband interacted and played with the dog, the easier it would be for Roy to accept him. However, the husband had to rigorously respond to any signs of aggression—of course, without punishing Roy physically. In addition, I mixed together several Bach flower remedies that the owners were to give him several times a day for a few days.

Three weeks later I heard from the owners. They reported that the dog now listened to both of them, but when he needed loving attention, he still preferred the wife.

Daily outings are just as important for a dog's psychological health as they are for its physical health.

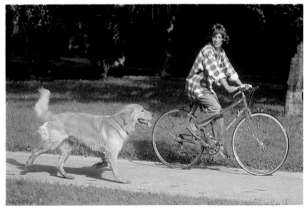

The Old Age of a Dog

TIP

If your dog suffers from degenerative joint disease and/or heart problems, make sure that it does not overexert itself. Several short walks a day would be better than one long walk.

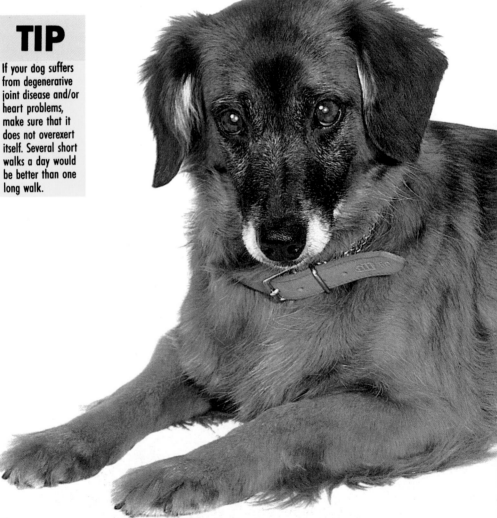

As a dog ages, it will seek much closer contact with the people in its life. Often a dog will take on characteristics that are similar to those of the owner, and sometimes dog and owner seem to look alike. The dog understands its master without a word being spoken and will detect emotions immediately. The countless walks they have taken together and the experiences they have shared have created an intimate relationship between the dog and its master. This is especially true when the owner is a senior citizen and they have grown old together.

Life Expectancy

The life span of a dog depends on several factors. A dog that has primarily lived inside and that has had a lot of human contact will usually live much longer than a dog that has spent its whole life outside, in a kennel or tied to a chain. So-called working dogs age faster than those that have had a life of leisure. The rule of thumb is that smaller breeds almost always live longer than larger breeds, and mixed breeds usually live longer than purebreds.

TIP

When you go on vacation, you should take an older dog's normal habits into account. If you leave the dog behind, make sure that the animal feels comfortable with the person who will care for it.

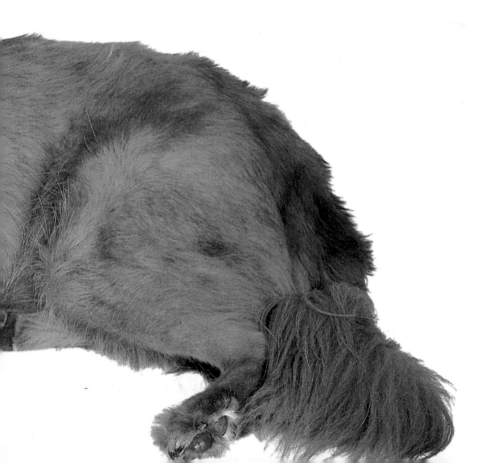

Top: This five-month-old boxer has many years to look forward to because boxers usually live ten to twelve years.

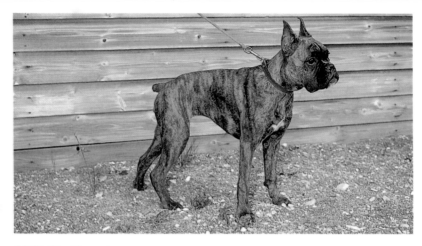

Middle: This female boxer is about five years old, in the prime of her life. Her age is roughly equivalent to that of a human who is thirty-five years old.

Bottom: Her body posture, graying fur, and the blue-gray color of her eyes immediately give away the age of this female boxer. She is about twelve years old.

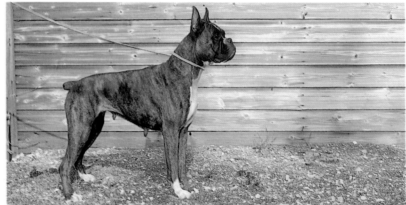

TIP

A dog with a hearing loss is in danger. This is particularly true for a dog living in a city. It should always be on a leash when out for a walk.

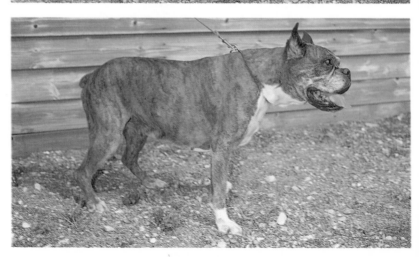

- Breeds with an average life span of ten to twelve years include: German shepherd, boxer, Newfoundland, Saint Bernard, Bernese mountain dog, Great Dane, and Doberman pinscher.
- Breeds with an average life span of thirteen to sixteen years include: poodle, dachshund, pug, terrier, Pekinese, collie, bullterrier, miniature and medium schnauzers, and spaniel.
- Breeds with a relatively long life span of sixteen to eighteen years include: spitz, miniature pinscher, and Lhasa apso.

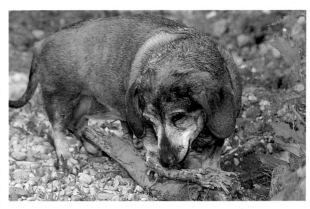

Physical Changes

The first physical changes are almost unnoticeable and take place when the dog is in the third stage of its life. The first gray hairs appear around the mouth. Later the whole area around the face and cheeks becomes gray. As is the case with people, the extent of graying varies widely. For dogs, the amount of gray hair depends on the breed or the mixture of breeds. In some animals, the whole head, the chest, and the front legs turn gray. Working dogs start to gray at a much earlier age than those that live indoors.

With increasing age, a dog's temperament begins to quiet down. The periods of intensive play grow shorter and occur less frequently. A dog that used to bark constantly and get excited about the slightest sound will now simply growl or let out a short bark. Some dogs develop rather odd and independent streaks, and many become somewhat stubborn, in a lovable way. When taking a walk, an older dog is much less inclined to engage in wild sprints and playful brawls. In earlier years, the dog would have pursued a cat with great joy; now the dog takes a few steps after the cat, but it's just for show. The older dog prefers to take its time, thoroughly sniffing each corner and under each bush in peace and quiet.

All activities become slower and quieter. The movements are not as powerful, and the body loses agility and seems more fragile. Particularly if the dog suffers from degenerative joint problems, it will walk stiffly and needs a little more time to get up and get going. We discuss how to use natural remedies for acute attacks of arthritis in "Case Histories," page 74.

As dogs get older some of their senses begin to diminish. In most cases, it is their eyesight that begins to fail first. But dogs are animals with a very well developed sense of smell. They are really "nose" animals, and poor eyesight doesn't significantly interfere with the quality of their lives. However, the situation is different when older dogs begin to lose some of their hearing.

As soon as you notice that your dog's hearing is changing, make sure that you

Even in its old age, a dachshund can still be a "real" dog. Much of its sense of smell remains intact, which means that the dog can do what it likes best: checking out the neighborhood—something every self-respecting dog must be able to do.

TIP

With increasing age the older dog begins to sleep much, much more. Do not mistake this for a form of withdrawal. Loving attention when he is awake is as important as when he was younger.

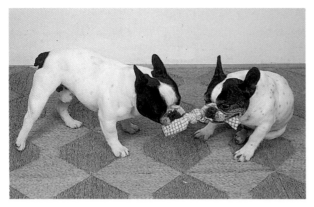

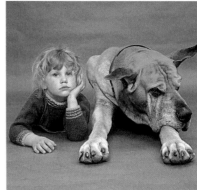

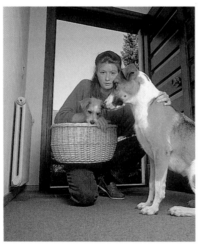

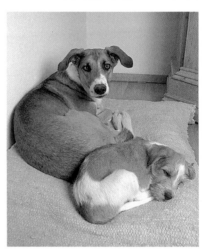

Upper left: In general, an older dog has a difficult time accepting a four-legged newcomer.

Upper right: Young children often bother an older dog. When this is the case, the dog will make its lack of interest clear.

Lower left: If you bring a young dog into the house, make sure you give the senior dog enough time to adjust.

Lower right: Sometimes a real friendship develops between an older dog and a newcomer. Here the old dog even allows the little one to sleep on its blanket.

accompany every command with a clear hand signal. In a short period of time, your dog will obey commands based on your hand signals.

Only the sense of smell remains intact in old age. But even if the sense of smell becomes less intense, enough remains for the dog to safely negotiate around its "fragrant" environment. Even if a dog is totally blind and deaf, it will recognize every member of its family immediately with the help of its nose. Highly scented or constantly changing perfumes might confuse the dog, but only for a moment.

Psychological Problems

An old dog has an increasingly difficult time adjusting to changes in its environment. Of course, the ability to adjust will depend on whether those changes alter the structure of its family or if its physical surroundings are changing. For instance, a dog might be excited for a while when the family moves to a different location or goes on a vacation. However, those situations are quite different from that faced by an old dog who loses a significant member of his "pack," which might cause a severe psychological shock, including true depression. Such a traumatic event might cause an preexisting age-related illness to worsen so rapidly that the dog dies in a very short time. From a medical point of view, saying that the dog died of a "broken heart" is very close to the truth. Fortunately many people are patient enough to help such an old dog get used to a new or changed home.

Anyone who wants to adopt an older dog that has lost its master should try to learn as much as possible about the life and habits that the dog experienced in its former home. What are the dog's eating and drinking habits? When does it get up in the morning? When was it usually taken for a walk? What are its likes and dislikes? The more the new owner honors these habits, the easier it will be for the dog to get used to the change. For example, if the former owner used the command "Come," but the new owner uses the command "Here," the new owner should not be surprised if the dog does not obey.

Bringing some of the dog's own belongings to the new place, such as its bed, blanket, a few toys, leash, and food

TIP

Start now to have your veterinarian check your dog twice a year.

Susceptibility to Illness and Nutrition

As is the case with an older person, the body of an aging dog begins to slow down. This means that the dog should eat a much lighter diet, including more oats, rice, and vegetables and less meat. Chicken, fish, and lean meat are more important than large portions of fatty meats. A low-salt diet will be helpful since an older dog may develop heart and kidney problems. The commercial diet foods on the market work very well.

Because older dogs often have a diminished sense of thirst, you need to make sure that your dog gets enough to drink.

Some dogs become constipated in old age. If that is the case, add paraffin oil and bulk (such as wheat germ) to your dog's food. Degenerative processes, such as arthritis, may affect an aging dog's joints. Arthritis is a typical problem for older dogs; only a few dogs escape it. Slipped disks are frequently a problem, particularly for dachshunds.

You can find some special recipes in "Diet for a Sick Dog" pages 86 and 87.

The increased tendency of older dogs to get tumors is another source of concern. Tumors can become malignant if not detected early enough.

A female dog that has not had her uterus removed is more susceptible to breast cancer than one who no longer has her uterus. Since a female's nipples grow larger after each litter, you might consider removing the uterus as a preventative measure. Examine an older female's nipples often in order to ensure early detection.

In "Case Histories," I have listed what you can do to treat old-age illnesses and included information about how to strengthen an old dog's overall physical condition.

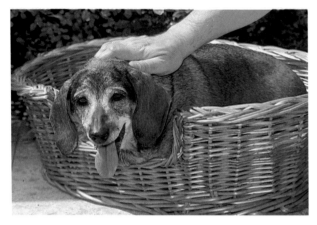

death. Personally, I believe that a dog has the right to experience its death and to die naturally. But putting a dog down should always be an option if prolonging the dog's life would mean that the dog has to endure pain and suffering. The quick prick from the needle is the only thing that the dog will feel if the veterinarian euthanizes the animal, and death occurs in a few seconds. If you decide to let the dog die naturally, Bach flower remedies can make the journey much easier. In most cases, however, the dog will die peacefully in its sleep.

Regardless of which choice you make, you should not leave your dog alone, no matter how painful it may be for you to witness its death. Your presence, your gentle stroking, and soft voice will make this final moment free from fear and anguish. Many veterinarians are more than willing to come to your house for this service because they know that a trip to the office is stressful and often creates fear. Allowing the dog to die in familiar surroundings is better for everyone.

Most older dogs will now spend more time in their favorite sleeping or resting place. But human attention should never be reduced—it might traumatize the dog.

and water dishes, helps make the change easier. The familiar scent of those things can be an invaluable psychological support in an otherwise strange surrounding.

The Last Good-Bye

Inevitably, the day will arrive when the owner must say a final good-bye to a dog that faithfully shared its life with him. More often than not the owner must face the decision of whether to have the dog put to sleep or to let the dog die a natural

When it's all over, you may want to bury your dog in your backyard, provided that your local area permits such a burial and providing that your dog isn't too big. Many animal shelters are willing to cremate your dog for a minimal fee. Of course, pet cemeteries are also available.

The Most Frequently Occurring Illnesses

Recognizable Symptoms	Possible Reasons	What You Can Do	See Your Veterinarian If
Discharge from the eye, sometimes accompanied by sensitivity to light; gray discoloration of the eyes; clouded pupils	Conjunctivitis; foreign object; injury to the cornea; gray or blue-green cataract or age-related blindness	Use cool compresses with chamomile; give *Euphrasia* 4 × several times a day; for gray cataracts, give Conjunctiva drops twice a day	No improvement within two days; foreign object or injury cannot be discounted
Yellow or watery discharge from the nose; frequent, severe sneezing	Foreign object in the nose; tumor	Inhalation with chamomile tea; in case of injury, give Traumeel tablets	Always, to find the cause
Coughing, increased or difficult breathing	Heart problems; tumor; less likely, parasites	Take temperature; inhalation with coltsfoot and chamomile tea	Always, to find the cause
Black deposits in the ears; foul odor; sensitivity to touch at the base of the ear; severe swelling; frequent scratching and head shaking, itching; hearing seems impaired	Ear-mite infection; ear infection (usually in dogs with floppy ears); age-related deafness; bloody ear	Apply oxygenated olive or calendula oil in the ear several times a day and massage the base of the ear	No improvement within one week; condition worsens; severe swelling
Black or white deposits on the fur; bare skin patches; severe scratching (itching); boils or hard bumps under the skin	Parasite infestation (fleas, lice, mites); skin fungus; hormone imbalance; problems with internal organs; tumor; fat boils; less likely, abscess	For fleas, use flea powder; give vitamin B and garlic; to bring abscess to a head, use *hepar sulfuris* 8 × several times a day; to heal an abscess, give *hepar sulfuris* 12 ×	No parasite detected; condition worsens; skin infection; always in cases of boils and hardened
Rapid weight loss; general weakness; unusual drinking and eating habits	Tumor; disease of internal organ or metabolism; old-age heart problems; less likely, parasites	Take temperature; deworm regularly; add vitamin B to food	Always, to find the cause
Boils, swellings, or inflammation in the area of the rectum; dog slides over the ground on its behind (itching); discharge from genitalia	Clogged anal glands; tumor; acute or chronic problems of the genitalia	Cool chamomile compresses; deworming regularly	No improvement within five days; problem recurs several times; boils or hard bumps; infections; always with discharge
Obvious effort when sitting down, lying down, getting up, or lifting leg; stiff, slow gait; some lameness	Arthritis or spondylitis (degenerative disease of the joints or spine); heart problem; injury to a limb	Cold or warm compresses (see what works best); give Traumeel pills several times a day; feed a lot of cartilage and gelatin	Lameness occurs frequently; dog can't move; dislocated joint; ligament problems or fracture suspected; foreign object suspected; in case of large bites
Diarrhea; loud rumbling noises in the intestines	Chronic problems in the digestive system or kidneys; spoiled food or poison; intestinal parasites	Take temperature; give only chamomile or black tea pills for twenty-four hours, follow with a light diet; give Kaopectate and *Echinacea*	Repeated diarrhea with other symptoms; poisoning suspected; no improvement for three days; temperature above 103°F (39.5°C) or below 100.5°F (38°C)
Vomiting	Chronic problems in the digestive system or kidneys; spoiled food or poison; ingested foreign object; intestinal parasites	Take temperature; give only peppermint tea pills for twenty-four hours, follow with a light diet; give *Nux vomica* 6 × and *Echinacea*	Poisoning or foreign object; additional symptoms appear; no improvement within three days; temperature above 103°F (39.5°C) or below 100.5°F (38°C)

Case Histories from My Practice

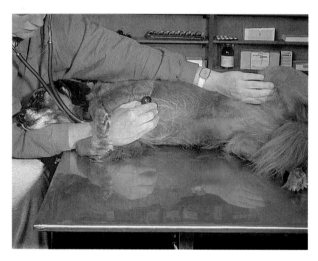

In order to detect heart problems, we use a stethoscope to examine the dog. We use the artery on the inside of the thigh to take a dog's pulse.

The Aging Heart

As with a person, a dog's heart begins to weaken as it grows older. Symptoms and complaints differ from one dog to another. If we detect heart problems early, we can usually prevent severe problems, and in that case, the dog can maintain the quality of its life. Unfortunately, the symptoms of heart disease are so varied that owners often don't recognize them for a long time.

In the case of Tilo, a twelve-year-old female terrier, her symptoms first suggested a psychological behavioral problem or an illness of the urinary tract. Tilo had never been sick a day in her entire life and had never before had an "accident." However, during the last three days, she had several accidents. Without any indication that she needed to go outside, she urinated in her bed. Her owners, an elderly couple, came to me for advice. The three of us suspected that she had a bladder infection, and they had brought a urine specimen with them. But the test turned out to be completely normal. A thorough examination showed that she had a very weak and irregular pulse. I explained to Tilo's owners that such a weakness is worse at night and that she was probably wetting her bed because heart and kidney functions were so closely related. I gave them a prescription for a plant extract to strengthen Tilo's heart and rid her system of accumulated fluids (edema). Since we have no cure for age-related weakness of the heart, I made sure that the owners understood the importance of giving Tilo her medication daily for the rest of her life.

Only three days later, Tilo's owners called and reported that the nightly accidents had stopped and the dog was much more lively. Unfortunately, Jessy, a ten-year-old mixed breed was a different case. She was in poor shape when her owner brought her to my office. Her heart was so weak that I feared death was imminent. Her pulse was irregular and very slow. When I listened to her heart, I

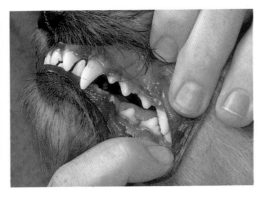 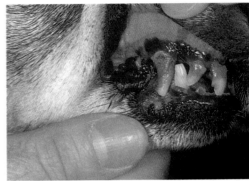

detected a major edema in her lungs. This was the reason for her labored breathing.

In addition to Bach flower remedy, I prescribed a complex herbal remedy to rid her of the excess fluid and to support and strengthen her circulatory system and heart. I also did acupuncture at points that respond best in emergency situations. After the threat to her life had subsided, I discussed a special diet plan with Jessy's owner and gave her a remedy consisting of several different types of herbs that the dog was to take every twelve hours.

A few days later, I listened to Jessy's heart and lungs again. Her pulse was much more normal, and I couldn't detect any lung sounds that would indicate edema. But since we can't cure an "old heart" with conventional or natural remedies, Jessy would have to continue taking the medication that had given her such relief.

Weak Kidneys

Kidneys also become less efficient in old age. Often owners don't recognize this condition until rather late because the typical symptoms, irregular drinking and urinating behaviors, are easy to overlook. Obvious signs are loss of appetite, vomiting, and weight loss. But these are signs of an advanced illness. Deteriorating teeth and chronically inflamed gums can disguise a developing or existing kidney problem. Complete kidney failure ends up poisoning the body because the metabolic wastes cannot be washed out of the system.

Fortunately, Arthos, a twelve-year-old male chow chow, was not even close to kidney failure. However, his owner had noticed that the dog was losing weight and drinking much more frequently than in the recent past. He was also vomiting frequently. A thorough examination showed kidney enlargement, a rough and dull coat, inflamed gums, and a foul-smelling breath. We extracted blood from a vein on his front leg and used part of it to do a quick kidney test in my office. I sent the rest to a laboratory for more thorough testing. As expected, the test results confirmed my diagnosis of chronic kidney disease. We started intravenous fluids to give Arthos some relief from the symptoms of the accumulated toxins and to prevent dehydration. In addition, I gave him an injection con-

Tarter accumulating along the gum line (right) usually causes gingivitis (left). However, chronic gingivitis may also be a sign of kidney problems or of internal diseases.

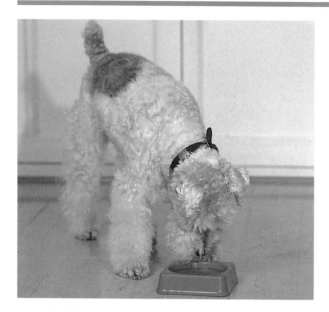

check the function of the kidneys and to react quickly to a possible decrease in kidney function.

Dachshund Paralysis

Contrary to popular belief, dachshund paralysis does not only affect dachshunds. It can also affect other dogs that have short legs or are built with a disproportionately long back. Dachshund paralysis is nothing more than a case of slipped disks. The center of the vertebra slips out of the soft outer tissue and pushes on the nerves in the spinal column. The nerve damage results in lameness, the severity of which varies. The part of the body that is affected depends on the position of the slipped disk. In particularly severe cases, surgery is the only effective treatment.

Fritz, a ten-year-old male dachshund, was more than well fed. Before his owner brought him to my office, Fritz had already had three episodes of paralysis, twice in the legs and once in the tail. The X rays the owner brought with him clearly showed arthritis of the small vertebrae. The owner thought that Fritz had been suffering from back pain for the past few days and that he also was having difficulty moving his tail.

When I started to examine him, I immediately noticed that the muscles of his back were as hard as a board. When I moved my fingers down his spine, Fritz seemed to cringe several times. As his owner had observed, the dog was unable to lift or move his tail, and his leg reflexes were very weak.

You can buy the Indian kidney tea used to treat dogs suffering from kidney problems and other ailments.

taining several different herb extracts to help him eliminate excess fluids and to support the kidneys. I sent the owner home with a similar preparation in pill form. The chow chow was take the pill and Indian kidney tea orally. As a general support and to strengthen all body functions, I gave the dog an injection of an organ preparation combined with vitamins. I removed the tartar and suggested that the owner apply disinfectant daily to the dog's teeth to treat his gingivitis. We also designed a strict kidney diet for the dog.

After a week, I repeated the office kidney test. Although all the values had greatly improved, they were still not back to normal. We continued the treatment as before. A week later, the next test showed that everything was back to normal, and I discontinued the injections. However, Arthos continued to take the oral medication, and he remained on the diet. Arthos came to my office every two months for blood tests, the only way to

Cancer

Cancer is a fatal disease for dogs as well as for people. Many older dogs develop tumors that can turn into cancer. Most of the tumors in dogs develop in the intestinal tract or in or on the genital organs, but tumors can appear in any part of the body. We can only determine whether or not a tumor is cancerous by examining a tiny piece of the tumor itself. If a tumor is malignant, the prognosis depends on which organ is involved, on whether the tumor has metastasized, and if it has, on how far it has spread. The age and the general condition of the dog play an important role.

We cannot cure cancer. However, we have several cancer therapies that often slow down the growth and can give an animal with cancer many years of happy life. However, good results depend on detecting the cancer early.

We can easily combine natural treatment methods with conventional treatment to make conventional treatments much easier for the dog. However, if the animal is in a lot of pain or is suffering in other ways, the owner should consider having it put to sleep, as difficult and painful as that decision might be.

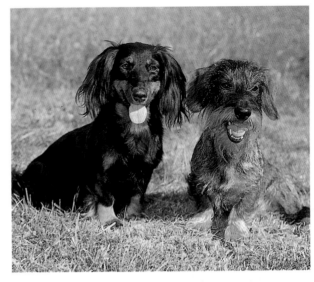

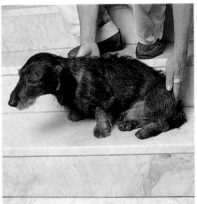

Above: The term "Dachshund paralysis"—a problem found primarily in dachshunds because of their long back and long legs—does by no means imply that only dachshunds are afflicted with this problem.

Left: A dachshund—because of the sensitive disks in the spine—should never walk up a flight of stairs by himself, but as a matter of course, should always be carried.

I treated the dog with acupuncture every third day. In addition, I used magnet therapy each time the dog came to my office. I also gave him an injection of a high dose of vitamin B combined with a homeopathic medication to provide relief for the nerves and to strengthen his overall physical condition. Both medications were also given orally at home.

Since every ounce of extra weight constitutes an additional burden for the spine, I strongly suggested that the owner put Fritz on a weight-loss diet.

In only one day, Fritz's back was much less sensitive to the touch, and he seemed much livelier. After four more days, he was able to move his tail normally and seemed to be free of pain. Fritz received a total of ten treatments, and I repeated the whole program every six months as a preventative measure.

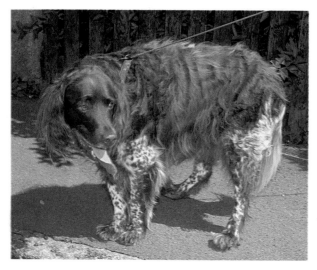

the dog an injection of ophidian extract and vitamins. In addition, I prescribed drops of ophidian extract and a homeopathic remedy to be taken orally. The owner gave these and a gelatin preparation to the dog several times a day.

Two days later, I put three leeches on both of Eywong's hip joints to reduce the pain as quickly as possible. Only one day later, Eywong was able to sit down and get up again without any appreciable evidence of pain. After six treatments, the dog had mobility in all joints again. As a preventative measure, we have treated Eywong with the same therapeutic regimen every six months. He is now in the best of health.

You can easily detect severe changes in the joints of the shoulders, knees, and hips just by looking at the dog's posture.

Arthritis

Typically, arthritis is a sign of aging. Large breeds, such as Saint Bernards, large schnauzers, and Great Danes, are particularly prone to arthritis of the large joints in the hip and shoulder and of the joints in the spine.

This was true for Eywong, a large eleven-year-old schnauzer. He had a lot of pain in his joints. His owner told me that the dog was having an increasingly difficult time getting up and lying down. She said Eywong required some time to start moving in the morning, and for a week his right hind leg had been lame.

A thorough examination of the large and slightly overweight dog showed a painful reduction of mobility in both hip joints. Since he had put on extra weight, his joints suffered even more stress. I was able to convince Eywong's owner to start him on a weight-loss diet immediately. I also put together an acupuncture regimen that I administered once a week. After each acupuncture treatment, I gave

General Strengthening Protocol

We have several natural healing methods that can delay age-related illnesses and slow down those that have already begun. Thus, it makes sense to treat your old dog to a regular program aimed at strengthening its general condition, even though your dog has no acute illness.

His owner brought ten-year-old Sultan to my office to do just that. This large dog, a mix of German shepherd and Great Dane, had been suffering from pain in his hip joints for the last year. The pain was the result of a rather severe case of arthritis. The owner told me that he seemed to be rather tired lately and did not do well in hot weather.

A thorough examination showed that his heart had grown rather weak. The movement of his right hip joint was limited and obviously painful. In addition, we had to immediately remove a thick layer of tartar covering his molars.

I prescribed a heart tonic that he was to take daily for the rest of his life to stimulate regeneration throughout his body. I treated the arthritis and the pain in his hips with weekly magnet therapy, applications of leeches, and injections of ophidian extract. The treatment continued for eight weeks. Sultan seemed much more lively and enjoyed his daily walks once more. His owner was so satisfied with the results that she brought him back six months later for another set of treatments.

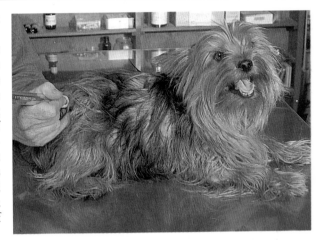

Acupuncture has been a very effective treatment for dogs with degenerative diseases.

Maintaining Good Health

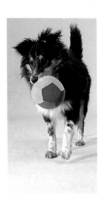

A healthy dog is happy, loves to go for walks, and loves to play.

A healthy dog has a shiny coat and looks at the world around it with sparkling-clear eyes. Its mouth, nose, eyes, ears, and anus are clean. It greets an invitation to go for a walk with great enthusiasm. A healthy dog also has a hearty appetite.

A dog's health depends on an appropriate environment and good care. This includes training, praise, and a loving touch, as well as a safe and clean place for sleeping and proper nutrition.

Good hygiene is also important. Don't forget to:

● Check every four months to make sure tartar hasn't accumulated on the gum line of the teeth. If it has, have a veterinarian or practitioner remove it.

● Let your dog have something to chew on. This helps prevent tartar buildup and massages the gums.

● Clean your dog's teeth once a week with a soft toothbrush and a special canine toothpaste.

● In general, daily walking keeps a dog's claws at their proper length, but if that is not the case, you must clip them. Clip the fifth claw regularly.

● During the winter months, apply a petroleum jelly to the pads of the dog's feet to protect them from the salt used to melt snow and ice.   •

● If necessary, remove any mud that has hardened between the toes.

● When it rains, dry the dog's coat when it comes inside, to prevent colds.

● When the weather is extremely hot, don't take your dog for a walk at noon. Just like many people, dogs don't do well in strong sunlight.

● On hot days, don't let your dog run with you when you are riding your bike.

● If your dog has long, floppy ears, clean them once a week with a paper towel and baby oil. Be careful! Cotton-covered sticks can puncture the eardrums.

● If a discharge appears in the corners of the eyes, use a cleansing tissue to remove the discharge. Use chamomile tea to wash away a crusty buildup.

● Brush a dog that has long fur once a day.

● Brush short-haired breeds now and then. They enjoy the special and loving attention.

● As you brush your dog, look for fleas, ticks, etc. Use flea powder when necessary.

● Help your dog get used to being brushed while it is still a puppy.

● Only give your dog a bath when it smells bad or is dirty. Use only dog shampoo.

● Make sure that you thoroughly dry your dog after you bathe it.

● Do not bathe puppies until they are at least six months old.

● A healthy dog is happy, loves to go for walks, and loves to play.

Health Checklist

Signs of Health	Signs of Problems or Illness	Possible Reasons	Special Tips
Eyes are clear, no discharge; thin fold in corner of the eye not visible	Discharge from the eye; eyes gummed up or lids swollen; thin fold in the corner of the eye visible; eyes red or very pale; pupils with a gray or blue tint, clouded over	Conjunctivitis; tear ducts are too narrow; viral infection; stress; tiredness; severe parasite infestation; gray cataracts; if conjunctiva is pale, possibility of heart or liver problems	Gray or "old age" cataract; in very old dogs, almost normal
Tip of nose dry or slightly moist, no discharge, no crusts, not gummed up; breathing is even, regular, and quiet	Nose gummed up or producing yellow discharge; sniveling, loud breathing, or frequent sneezing	Nose is too small and narrow (in Pekinese, boxer, pug breeds); viral infection (distemper); allergies; sensitivity to odors; tumors; stress	In case of stress or high fever, panting and clear discharge is normal; in old dogs, dripping nose is a sign of stress
Pink gums; teeth without heavy plaque or discoloring	Pale to whitish or inflamed gums; swollen and bleeding gums; severe discoloration of teeth with brown deposits on the gum line	Severe parasite infestation; problems with internal organs; gingivitis; plaque; damaged tooth enamel after distemper infection	Gums often swollen as permanent teeth come in; lost or broken teeth due to accident or chewing on stones; in old dogs, missing teeth are normal
Ear canal clean and odor free; no sensitivity to touch at the base of ear; no frequent scratching that might indicate itching	Black deposits or crusts in the ear canal; discharge or foul odor; base of ear sensitive to touch; obvious frequent scratching; swellings	Inflammation of the ear canal, usually caused by long, floppy ear or ear-mite infection; bloody ear	Cocker spaniels most prone to ear infections because long, furry ears prevent proper exposure to air
Coat shiny and clean; long hair not matted; no bare patches; no evidence of black or white deposits	Dull, dry, or matted fur; black or white deposits in the fur; bare skin, discolored or not; constantly scratching, chewing, or licking (itching); obvious small lumps under the skin	Long-standing general illnesses; parasites; round, bare skin; skin fungus; hormone imbalance; allergies or psychological problems; tumors	Bare, callused skin on legs or elbows from sleeping is normal; fur of old dogs often looks dull; dogs that have not been neutered often have hormone imbalances
Belly soft and supple; no resistance to pressure; rounded shape; no lumps detectable under the skin of the belly; in females, nipples are soft and not enlarged; in females, hard breasts	Tight, swollen pot belly or pear-shaped drooping belly; resistance to slight pressure; audible sounds from the intestines; abdominal wall hard	Parasite infestation of the intestines (usually spool worms and tapeworms); other intestinal infections; liver and heart problems; poorly functioning pancreas; tumors	Tumors; very prevalent in old dogs
Anus area clean without crusts or inflammation; closed sphincter muscle; no discharge from genital organs	Anus crusted over, red, and swollen; open and drooping sphincter muscle; immobile tail; yellow discharge from the penis or vagina	Diarrhea and/or intestinal parasites; blocked, inflamed anal glands; paralysis; prostate problems; vaginitis; uterus infection; inflammation of the foreskin	Inflammation of vagina or foreskin, from distemper infection; uterus infection, particularly in old females
Dog reacts spontaneously to external stimuli	Listlessness, apathy; fearfulness; overly anxious or aggressive	Behavior problems; lack of or incorrect training	Reactions of old dogs often slow; deafness or blindness

Caring For an Ill Dog

TIP

You can use a child's or a digital thermometer to take a dog's thermometer because both have a narrow tip.

A sick dog needs loving care from the person it trusts most. This section contains many tips to help you care for your sick or injured animal at home. It also has suggestions to help you carry out the instructions your veterinarian or practitioner gives. You can easily and safely use the "gentle" methods discussed here (such as how to make a compress, poultice, or initiate inhalation) along with the therapy provided by your veterinarian or practitioner. However, you should always inform your veterinarian or practitioner of what you intend to do at home.

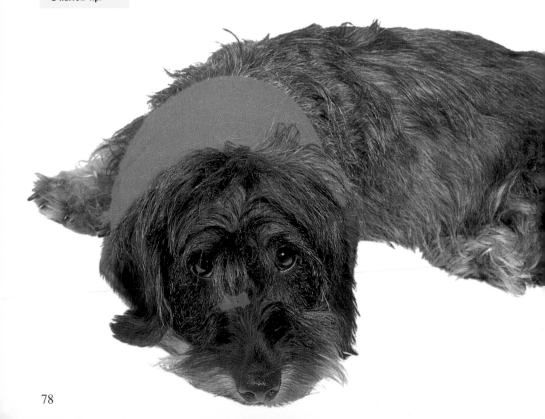

Taking Temperature

No dog likes having its temperature taken, but sometimes that is just what you need to do; and on occasion, you need to do it not once but twice a day. This is the only way to keep track of how an illness is progressing or improving. In addition, many infectious diseases have a very characteristic fever curve. Thus, a record of your dog's temperature often makes it much easier to correctly diagnose the illness.

A dog's normal temperature is between 101°F (38.3°C) and 102°F (39°C). However, simply getting excited, for instance by having its temperature taken, may raise a dog's normal temperature. A temperature of 106°F (41°C) is life-threatening. On the other hand, a slightly elevated temperature is not critical. However, a body temperature of less than 100.5°F (38°C) is a sign that your dog is seriously ill.

Simply touching your dog in order to determine if it has fever won't do. Contrary to popular belief, you cannot tell if a dog's temperature is normal or elevated by whether or not its nose is wet or dry or by whether its ears or pads are cold. In addition, the way your dog behaves is not a sure sign of its temperature. Young dogs are able to deal with fevers; they are often still playing with a temperature of 104°F (40°C).

When getting ready to take your dog's temperature, dip the tip of the thermometer in oil and then insert it about ¾ in (2cm) deep in the rectum. Leave it in place for about two minutes.

Throughout the procedure, talk to your dog with a soothing, quiet voice. If you have a very self-confident or unpredictable dog, you might need to use a muzzle or to wrap a bandage or towel around its mouth. Not many dogs will voluntarily remain still for two minutes, so be careful and watch out!

Holding a Puppy

Hold the puppy on your lap and turn it on its back so that it is against your stomach. With one hand, reach between its front legs and hold on to the paws of the hind legs. Depending on whether or not your dog is holding still, you might want to wedge its head between your arm and body or just let its head rest against you. With your other hand, move the tail to one side and insert the thermometer. If the puppy is too big for your lap, you'll need another person to help hold it on the floor, the same way you would if it were on your lap.

Holding an Adult Dog

If your dog is small, you can use the same method you would with a puppy, but if it is bigger than a dachshund, you'll need a second person to help you. Choose someone the dog already knows. Let the dog stand up. Your helper should put one arm around the dog's chest and, with the other hand, reach under and around the dog's neck. You can then insert the thermometer. Of course, you can also take a dog's temperature when it is lying down. In that case, your helper should kneel behind the dog and put one arm under the dog's head so that he can hold the

TIP

You can use a conventional thermometer to take a dog's temperature. Hold it in place for at least two minutes, less if you use a digital thermometer.

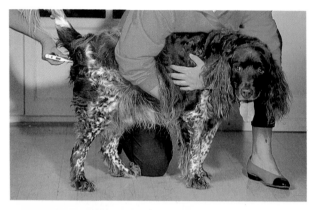

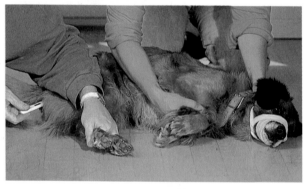

Make sure that the food dish and the water bowl are close by. In many cases, you might want to keep the bed warm. For more information, check "Treatment with Dry, Warm Heat," page 85.

Inhalations

We use inhalations for illnesses involving the upper respiratory tract and the lungs. Inhalation may shorten the length of an illness, and most dogs seem to enjoy the procedure. However, under no circumstances should you add essential oils to inhalations. The fragrance, which even people find very strong, would be too intense for your dog's nose, which is much more sensitive than yours. You'll find suitable additives listed in "Natural Healing Remedies in Your Medicine Cabinet," pages 16 and 17 .

Top: If you have a large dog, you'll need help taking its temperature. One person holds the dog so that it cannot run away, and the other inserts the thermometer.

Below: If the animal cannot or will not stand up, take its temperature while it is lying down. Even if the dog is lying down, you'll need two people for a large dog.

front legs. He places the other hand on the dog's chest or holds the hind legs so that you can insert the thermometer.

The Sickbed

If your dog is so sick that it can't stand up or move around on its own, you should prepare a comfortable and proper "sickbed." If possible, choose a place where your dog can see you.

Start with a rubber mat or plastic bag. Place a thick layer of newspaper on the mat or bag and a comfortable blanket or a large towel on top of the newspaper.

You may use a whole room, such as your bathroom, for a steam bath. Fill several wide bowls or your bathtub with hot water. However, if your dog is not too big, you might want to set the dog on your lap, put a big towel over your head, and place the steaming bowl between your knees. Of course, you need to be careful that you don't scald the dog or yourself with the hot water.

You can also place a small dog in a wicker cat carrier that has a lid. Put the carrier (with the lid closed) on an upside-down stool in such a way that you can slide a bowl of steaming hot water under it. To increase the intensity of the steam, you might want to place a large towel or blanket over the carrier.

Allow the dog to stay in the carrier for at least five minutes—better yet, fifteen minutes. Do this two or three times a day. And don't worry if you notice that the dog has a runny nose or a cough immediately after the steam bath. These are signs that the inhalation has been effective, loosening the congestion in the respiratory tract and lungs.

Force-feeding and Giving Medication

In most cases, a dog can't understand why it should obediently swallow the medicine that its owner tries to shove down its throat. The best way to give a dog fluids, such as tea, broth, or a medication diluted in water, is with a disposable syringe, minus the needle, of course. In most cases, you'll only need a 2ml syringe and a 20ml syringe. These should be part of the equipment you keep in your medicine cabinet.

Make sure that the liquid is free of lumps that might choke your dog. Place the dog on your lap, in the same position

as you would use to take its temperature, or stand over a dog that is sitting down. Hold his mouth closed with one hand and bend his head back. With the other hand, slide the syringe from the side into the space behind the dog's canines. Empty the syringe slowly into its mouth, pausing a few times as you do so. You can

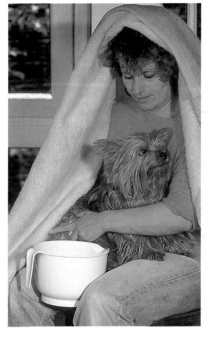

Left: The best way to use an inhalation with a small dog is to put the dog on your lap and sit with it under a blanket with a steaming bowl of water.

Below: Using a hot-water bottle to keep a sickbed warm might seem a bit cumbersome because you have to change the water in the bottle to keep the temperature constant. However, using a hot-water bottle means that you don't have to place the bed close to an electrical outlet.

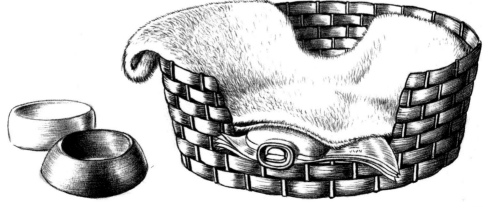

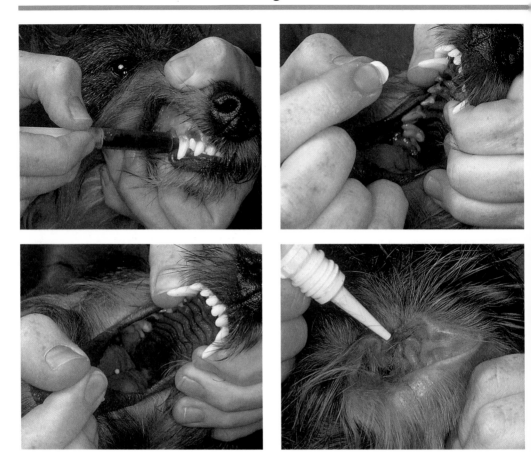

You can use a disposable syringe, without the needle, to administer fluids (above left). To give a pill, open the mouth (above right) and allow it to fall as far back as possible (below left). If your dog needs ear drops, don't insert the dropper into the ear canal (below right).

administer small amounts of liquid directly by pulling the lips away slightly.

If the dog resists, ask another person to help you by holding the dog in the manner just discussed. Your helper should stand with his back against a wall. This position makes it impossible for the dog to escape between the helper's legs.

If you cannot or should not dissolve a pill in water, you'll have to place it as far back in the throat as possible so that the dog cannot spit it out. Hold the dog's head back, as described for giving liquid medications, place the thumb and index finger of one hand behind the canine teeth between the upper and lower jaw. At the same time, place the middle finger of the other hand between the incisors and push the lower jaw down. Hold the medication between the thumb and index finger of the first hand. As soon as the dog's mouth is open, let the medication fall as far back in its throat as possible. Quickly close the jaws. If the dog does not swallow immediately, you can help by gently massaging the throat. Be very careful; this method can be dangerous if the dog is particularly stubborn. If this is the case, let your veterinarian or practitioner administer the medication.

Compresses and Poultices

In general, we distinguish between hot and cold, dry and wet compresses, and poultices. Dry compresses are easy to prepare using gel-filled "pillows" available at pharmacies. For the others, you need a cotton cloth, such as a dishcloth or a handkerchief, and a woolen cloth. You can cut up an old wool blanket or cut off the sleeve of an old sweater. Either of these will hold a compress in place. A compress should never be too tight. In general, dogs seem to be comforted by a compress or poultice. However, if your dog is fighting the whole procedure or becomes restless at any point, simply remove the cloth. A compress should always feel good. Never force one on your dog.

Throat Compress

A compress around the throat usually lessens the symptoms of a cold or an inflamed throat. Place a cotton cloth, not too wet or too cold, around the dog's neck and pull a wool sock, with the toe end cut off, over the dog's head. Leave the compress in place for ten to fifteen minutes. If you place a dry wool sock around the dog's neck after you remove the wet compress, you can increase the effectiveness of this treatment.

Compress for the Chest

If your dog suffers from bronchitis or pneumonia with only a slight fever, a chest compress is effective. This compress is not very different from a throat compress, but you place it on the chest. Keep the compress in place with a headband.

Body Compress

If your dog is suffering from a bellyache, a warm body or tummy compress is very soothing. But make sure that you check with your veterinarian or practitioner for advice, because some illnesses will get

A body compress is always warm, but it may be wet or dry.

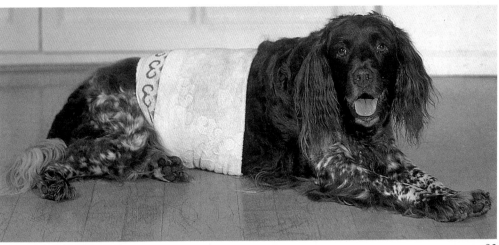

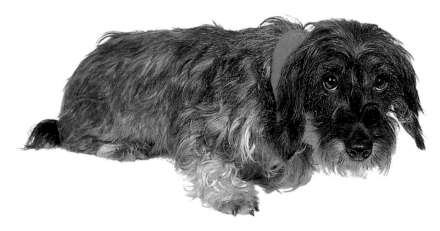

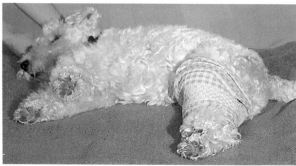

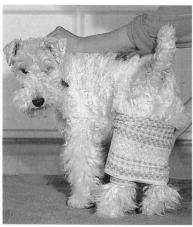

Top: A throat compress is always wet and cold.

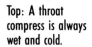

Right: Apply leg compresses, used to lower a fever, while the dog is standing.

Left: Since a dog cannot walk around with a leg compress on, let the dog lie on its side after you apply the compress.

worse if you apply a compress. In any case, a warm body compress is a wonderful method to treat your dog when its temperature is below normal. A body compress may be wet or dry. However, you should remove a warm, wet cloth after five or ten minutes because by then it has cooled down.

Leg Compresses

For ages, people have used leg compresses to lower high fevers. They work just as well for animals. Since a dog cannot move around during the procedure, you should stay with it and give it tender loving strokes.

Put a wet, cold cotton cloth between the dog's hind legs and then wrap it around both legs. Cover the legs with a wool blanket. Remove the compress after five minutes, dip the cotton cloth in cold water, and repeat the procedure.

Compress with Healing Earth

Compresses made with healing earth can speed up the healing process for wounds that are not doing well. They are also useful in healing abscesses and skin disorders. You can purchase healing earth at health-food stores. Mix the healing earth with warm water to create a thick consistency. Place the mixture between two single gauze pads, covering the affected area. Keep the compress in place by wrapping an old sock or a wool cloth around it. For best results, keep this compress in place for twenty minutes.

Cold Compresses

In the event of a sprain, a localized injury, or an inflammation, cold compresses usually bring quick relief. Place a folded, cold, wet cloth or an ice bag over the affected area. Remove the compress after a few minutes and repeat the procedure after a short rest.

Treatment with Dry, Warm Heat

Warmth, the most important prerequisite for all biological processes, also promotes healing. Heat stimulates the metabolism and increases the flow of blood in the area you apply it to. You can use dry heat treatment in different ways:

Infrared Light

Compared to other light sources, the warmth created by an infrared light penetrates relatively deep into the tissues, increasing circulation in the area exposed to it. Infrared-light therapy, however, creates considerable stress on the circulatory system, so very weak dogs or those with a weak circulatory system often are unable to tolerate it. Keep a close eye on your dog during the treatment. The dog must be able to move away from the lamp if it wants to.

If you are treating the total dog, for instance, to raise a body temperature that has fallen below the acceptable level or if the goal is to strengthen the overall condition, place the dog in its basket or put a small dog on your lap. Place the lamp about 20in (50cm) away from the dog. Use the lamp for ten to fifteen minutes. If the dog becomes restless, discontinue the treatment. You can use this whole-body treatment several times a day.

In case of arthritis or a cold, treat only the affected joint or the nose and sinuses. The distance between the dog and the lamp should be about 12in (30cm).

You can use infrared light to treat individual parts of the dog's body, or you can treat the whole body. Never leave your dog alone during treatment.

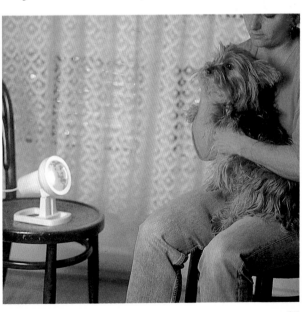

85

TIP

If your dog is seriously ill and has become very weak, you can use a disposable syringe to feed it baby food that is free of gluten and milk sugar and does not contain fruits or vegetables that could produce gas.

Diet for a

If your veterinarian or practitioner tells you that your dog needs to go on a diet, divide the food into small portions and feed it three or four times a day. We have not included measurements in the recipes for different diets since the amount of food will depend on the dog's size.

Diet for Stomach and Intestinal Problems

In general: Many dogs are like garbage disposals. They will eat anything and everything that comes their way when on a walk, and, unfortunately, some of what they eat does not agree with them. Their systems react with diarrhea or vomiting. In most cases, you can treat the problem with a one-day fast followed by a one-day diet. The same holds true for dogs that have eaten too much snow.

Menu I: Fish Fillet
Boil low-fat fish in plenty of water. Add a little instant oats and low-fat cottage cheese. Offer this to your dog at least four times a day. Instead of water give the dog a diluted tea made with black tea, chamomile, and peppermint.

Menu II: Chicken and Rice
Boil rice in plenty of water until it is sticky and forms clumps. Add well-cooked chicken and broth (remove fat first). You can substitute turkey or lamb for the chicken meat. Divide in small portions and feed your dog at least four times a day. To quench thirst, give your dog diluted tea as described in Menu I.

Diet for Constipation

In general: Constipation is a malady that often plagues older dogs. Don't permit your dog to chew bones, because this often causes constipation. Add a little paraffin oil to every meal. This will increase the movement of the food as well as the stool in the intestinal tract. Adding fiber to the food is also helpful. Make sure that everything is cut into small pieces because this makes food easier to digest.

Menu I: Lamb Stew
Mix the cooked meat with a small amount of raw beef liver, and a generous amount of raw oatmeal that has been thoroughly soaked, one tablespoon of olive oil, one cooked and pureed carrot, and a small amount of applesauce.

Menu II: Beef Liver and Oatmeal
Mix raw liver (cooked liver would cause even more constipation) with raw oats that have been thoroughly soaked. Add one tablespoon of oil and a small amount of dry, stale, cubed rye bread. A few herbs and a few drops of vegetable oil will add a delicious touch to this meal.

Diet for Weight Loss

In general: Unfortunately, many dogs tend to be overweight. While too much weight doesn't seem to be a problem for cats, dogs often have health problems when they are overweight. This is particularly true for those that tend to

Sick Dog

be prone to dachshund paralysis or to hip displacement. These dogs should not carry any extra weight.

Menu I: Giblets Stew
Mix cow udder, as available, and chicken stomachs and a little beef and boil all. Add plenty of cooked rice or millet and a few drops of vegetable oil.

Menu II: Colorful Polenta (cornmeal)
Boil a chicken and remove the bones. Boil the polenta in the broth until it is thick. Add the diced chicken, one diced carrot, and a small amount of low-fat cottage cheese.

Diet for Allergies and Skin Problems

In general: A dog with skin problems (often caused by allergies) should only eat lamb meat. In time, you may want to introduce chicken, turkey, and fish, making sure that the condition does not reappear. Carbohydrates should consist of gluten-free grains (such as millet, buckwheat, rice, and corn). Add borage oil, evening primrose oil, garlic, and vitamin B (in the form of brewer's yeast) to the food.

Menu I: Lamb with Buckwheat
Boil lamb in a sufficient amount of water until done. Remove the meat and add buckwheat to the broth. Boil until you have a thick mush. Add a small amount of garlic, 1 teaspoon (5ml) of borage oil, and one grated carrot.

Menu II: Lamb Stew
Boil equal parts of lamb and innards in a sufficient amount of water until done. Remove the meat and add millet to the broth. Boil until you have a thick mush, then mix in the meat. Add a small amount of garlic, a ¼ teaspoon (1ml) of evening primrose oil, and one mashed carrot.

Diet for Strengthening

In general: A strengthening diet should consist of high-quality protein and fat. The diet also needs to be rich in vitamins, especially the vitamin B groups (such as those contained in brewer's yeast) because they increase the animal's appetite. This diet is very good for young, growing dogs. Give it to them at regular intervals while they are in an active growth period. However, this diet is also very important for dogs recovering from severe and prolonged illnesses.

Menu I: Meat Stew
Boil beef, udder, as available, chicken, and a small amount of beef or chicken hearts. Adjust the amount to your dog's taste. Add about two-thirds of the cooked meat to cooked noodles and raw or steamed carrots. Before serving, add high-quality vegetable oil (corn oil), parsley, and a small amount of garlic.

Menu II: Liver Stew
Mix equal parts of raw and cooked beef and calf liver. Add cottage cheese and about half of the cooked rice. Add a small amount of parsley or chives, a small amount of garlic, and the yoke of one egg.

Top left: To muzzle your dog, first place the loop of a bandage around its mouth.

Lower left: Tie the two ends underneath the chin and move them left and right, alongside its jaws.

Top right: Tie both ends behind its head.

Lower right: This is what a properly muzzled dog looks like. Sometimes you need to muzzle a dog to avoid being injured while you take care of it.

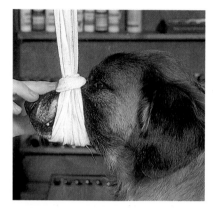

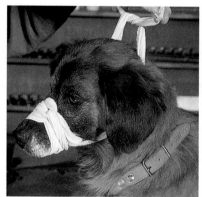

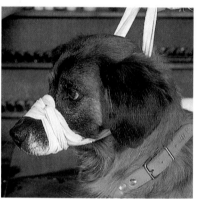

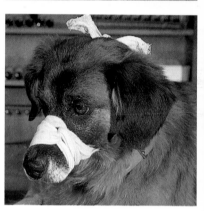

Place your hand next to the area you want treated. This gives you a way to monitor the heat absorbed by the skin. If you treat the dog's face, make sure that you cover each eye with two fingers. Expose the dog for about ten minutes, preferably several times a day.

Hot-Water Bottle

The hot-water bottle is still the easiest and safest way of providing warmth to an animal. The hot water in the bottle needs to be replaced frequently. The temperature of the water should never exceed 102°F (39°C). Wrap the bottle in a towel and place it so that it touches the dog's belly or upper body.

If your dog is too sick to move on its own, you must turn it over every ten to twenty minutes. Make sure you constantly check the dog's condition and the temperature of the bottle.

If you are caring for orphaned puppies, try to keep the temperature at a constant 100.5°F (38°C).

Electric Heating Pad

Because an electric heating pad is a steady source of heat, it is ideal for orphaned puppies that are in need of warmth. However, a heating pad is vulnerable to wetness and to a dog's claws and teeth. To avoid electrical shocks to you and the dog, carefully wrap the pad. Place it in a plastic bag and close the bag with adhesive tape. Wrap the bag in several thick layers of newspaper, and then wrap the whole package in a pillowcase or a large towel.

Keep the setting on high until the bed is thoroughly warm. No more than ten minutes later, adjust the temperature to the lowest setting.

Applying a Muzzle

If your dog tends to bite easily, you should put a muzzle on it before you attempt to treat it. Remember that severe pain or the shock from an accident can turn your usually docile dog into a dangerous, biting animal. Even if several people are present at the time, only the owner should put on the muzzle, because in extreme situations dogs will inevitably bite a stranger.

Use an elastic bandage or a wide piece of cloth to make a muzzle. Fold the bandage in half, forming a loop. Slip this loop over the dog's head in one quick motion and pull the ends together. Tie them under the chin and guide them alongside the jaws and behind the ears.

If you want to use this method to handle a dog that is frantically biting and snarling, hold a rolled-up sweater, a thick towel, or something similar in front of your hand and let the dog bite what you are holding before you try to muzzle it. But I must warn you that the dog is still dangerous and may bite you.

Bandaging

In most cases, applying a bandage to a dog is very difficult. Sometimes, however, it is necessary; for instance, when you need to cover a wound. You must tie the bandage tight enough that it won't come undone when the dog moves or pulls on it.

Bandaging a Front Leg

To bandage a paw you must have a tube bandage approximately the size of the dog's leg. Cut a piece of bandage about three times as long as the dog's leg, knotting one end. Pull the bandage over the paw as if it were a sock. Cut the bandage lengthwise on both sides just below the shoulder. Pull one end under the chest and forward between the legs, passing one leg, up to the back. Slip the other end up over the back.

Tie both ends together. Tie the ends that extend past the knot to the collar. The last step is to bend the knot at the bottom of the paw up and over and to secure it with adhesive tape so that the knot does not create pressure on the pad. You can also use adhesive tape to fasten the bandage around the elbow. Check to be sure that the bandage doesn't cut into the armpit. If it is too tight, cut the bandage on both sides a bit farther down, so that there is less of the "tube."

If the dog has a cut, you may need to create a pressure bandage by putting an elastic bandage around the leg. Before you use a pressure bandage, make sure that no foreign object (splinter or dirt) is in the wound. In addition, You need to cushion the space between the toes and pads with cotton.

TIP

In case of serious illness or injuries, do not leave your dog alone for more than two to three hours, which is also good advice for a dog younger than six months. If you are working, find a good neighbor or look for a dog-sitter.

Top: Use a tubular bandage to bandage a leg.

Middle: Pull the tubular bandage over the leg as if it were a sock.

Bottom: Tie the ends of the bandage together securely so that it will remain in place.

TIP

Pet shops carry special leather "shoes" to protect a dog's bandaged legs.

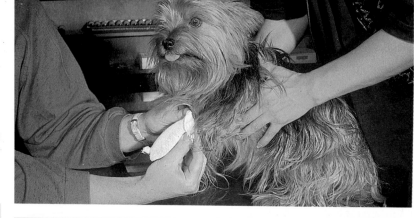

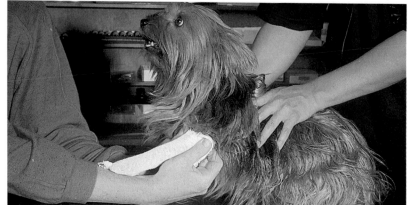

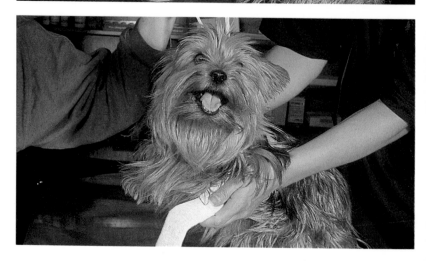

Bandage for a Hind Leg

Start with a tubular bandage that is 20 to 28in (50 to 70cm) long. Tie a knot in the end. Pull the bandage up and over the knee as you would a sock and fasten it as outlined above. Here, too, tie the ends to the collar.

Body Bandage

To bandage the body of a small dog, you need a large tubular bandage. For big dogs, you'll need to enlarge the neck of a T-shirt or use a man's undershirt. For a small dog, cut a piece of bandage twice the length of the dog's body. Cut the bandage in four places for the four legs, each about 1in (3cm) long. Pull the bandage over the dog's head and pull the legs through the holes, one at time. Pull the ends of the bandage up over the shoulder blades and tie them together. Check the leg openings. If they are too tight, enlarge them.

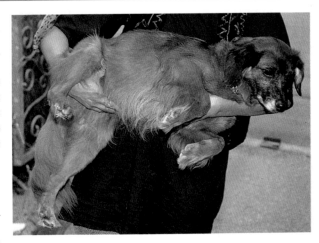

Bandaging the Tail

To bandage the tail, you need a small tubular bandage. Cut a piece that is about twice as long as the tail and tie a knot at one end. Pull the bandage over the tail, as you would a sock, and cut the bandage lengthwise on the right and left sides at the base of the tail. Tie the ends in a knot and move them along the back to the neck, fastening them around the collar.

You can use the "calf hold" to transport an injured dog, providing that the dog is not unconscious.

Top: The best way to transport an injured dog is on a blanket.

Middle: To transport a panicky dog, wrap a towel over its head, covering its eyes.

Bottom: Two people can use a blanket as a stretcher to transport an injured dog.

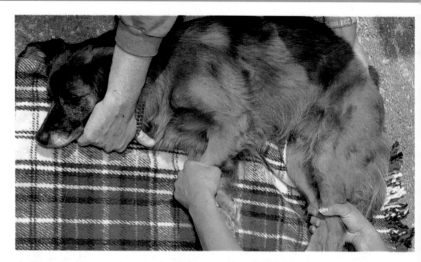

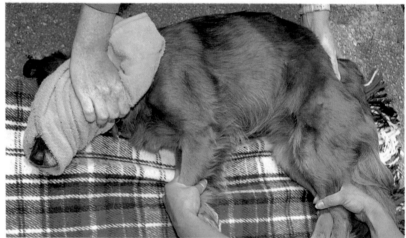

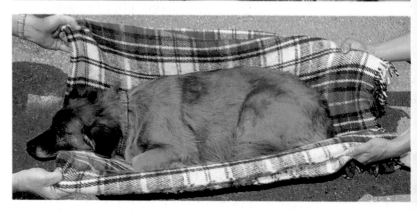

First Aid

What follows is a discussion of some of the accidents and injuries that are common to dogs, as well as tips on how to recognize them and suggestions on how to provide first aid for a seriously injured animal. Remember that after you have safely provided first aid, you must transport the animal immediately to a veterinarian or to a clinic.

What You Should Always Do

● Always give a few drops of Bach Flower Rescue Remedy to an injured dog.

● Call the veterinarian's office or the clinic to make sure that a qualified staff person will actually be there when you arrive. If surgery is necessary, the veterinarian can make the necessary preparations while you are transporting the dog.

Transporting the Sick Animal

Try not to transport an injured animal by yourself. If possible, bring another person along with you. Grab the skin of the animal at the neck and the back or the base of the tail and pull it onto a blanket that you have laid flat on the ground. Two people can carry the blanket as if it were a stretcher. This will prevent further injury from twisting or turning the dog's body. You can transport a smaller dog in a box. However, the box should be fairly narrow so that the animal doesn't move back and forth during the transport. If necessary, make the space inside the box smaller by placing a towel or blanket around the dog.

If you must handle an injured animal alone, use the "calf hold." Reach through the dog's front legs and place your hand on its chest. Reach through its hind legs and place your other hand on its stomach. Rest the dog's back against your stomach when carrying it. Carry an unconscious dog on its side. Ideally, its head should point slightly down, towards the ground. Pull the tongue forward and a little to the side so that the dog won't start to choke and so that if it vomits, the vomitus will only drain out of its mouth.

If the dog is conscious and panicky, wrap a towel around its head, covering its eyes. You may need to tie a towel around its mouth or make a muzzle.

Injuries

● *Fractures and Torn Ligaments*
You'll recognize a fracture by the dislocation of the limb or a portion of the limb. In addition, the animal cannot put any weight on the leg. Rib fractures are difficult to see. In most cases, the dog won't be able to get up or walks as if on eggs.

An injured ligament causes the affected joint to become very unstable. For that reason and because of the pain, the dog won't put any weight on the leg.

What to Do
If you must carry the animal, put one arm through the front leg and place your hand on its chest; support the body with the other hand by sliding your arm through its hind legs and

TIP

If you suspect that a dog has sustained internal injuries (for instance, from an accident), place the dog on a white sheet while you transport it to the veterinary clinic. The white sheet will reveal any vomit, urination, or bleeding.

TIP

In case of superficial injuries, disinfect the wound and apply a salve to start the healing process.

placing your other hand on the stomach.

If you suspect an internal fracture and the dog is unable to get up, put a muzzle on the dog to protect yourself. Then grab the skin at the neck and at the back and pull the dog onto a blanket. You can carry this as if it were a stretcher.

●*Cuts*

Most cuts are to the legs. In serious cases, for example, if the dog has been rolling in a lot of broken glass, it may have injuries all over its body, from head to toes. A cut is easy to recognize because the wound has a smooth edge and bleeds heavily.

What to Do?

Treat superficial cuts by disinfecting them. Then use a healing salve. Seek professional care immediately for wounds that are wide open and deep and in cases where you cannot be sure that there is no foreign object in the wound. If in doubt, obtain professional help.

●*Bites*

Most bite wounds are the result of fights between dogs. But a confrontation with a cat can have serious consequences, too. Although a cat's bite is usually small and inconspicuous, it may penetrate all the layers of the skin and enter a muscle.

Large bites are usually wide open with ragged edges. Surprisingly, these wounds don't bleed very much.

First

What to Do?

Examine your dog carefully after it has a fight with another dog. The neck, face, shoulder, and ears sustain the most injuries. Disinfect the surface of the wounds. If they are very deep and you not sure of the extent of the injury, see your veterinarian.

●*Foreign Objects in the Mouth or Throat*

Foreign objects frequently lodge in a dog's mouth or throat because the dog has been playing with them and chewing on them enthusiastically or because the dog gulped food down too hastily. When this occurs, a dog will get very anxious and restless, trying to remove what bothers it with a paw. The flow of saliva is very heavy, and the dog will refuse to let you look in its mouth. If the object interferes with breathing, the dog will start coughing and trying to vomit.

What to Do?

First, try to calm down your dog. Ask another person to hold the dog between his legs while you try to pry its mouth open by pulling the upper and lower jaws apart. Only the dog's owner should try to do this. If you are unable to remove whatever is stuck in the mouth or throat, seek professional help immediately.

●*Bee or Wasp Sting*

Sooner or later, every dog has a painful confrontation with a bee or wasp.

In general, this happens when the dog steps or rolls on the insect in the grass. The dog reacts to the burning sensation of the sting. A sting on a paw causes lameness. The dog will start to lick the paw ferociously. A sting on the head usually results in an impressive swelling. A sting inside the mouth or throat may lead to serious breathing problems and even death by suffocation.

What to Do?
Applying something cold to the sting is the easiest and most effective treatment for pain and swelling. Anything cold will do. You can place the paw in cold water or put an ice bag on it. You can make a cold, wet compress from a cold cloth. Give the dog Apis 4 × every four hours. This homeopathic remedy is effective in most cases. If your dog has been stung in the mouth or throat, give it ice-cold water to drink and immediately bring the dog to a clinic or your veterinarian.

● *Injuries from a Car Accident*
When a dog has sustained severe injuries on different parts of the body, it has usually been in a car accident.

What to Do?
Immediately transport your dog to a clinic or your veterinarian (see "How to Transport an Injured Dog"). You won't always be able to recognize internal bleeding, and simple shock can endanger a dog's life.

● *Heat Stroke*
On hot summer days, a dog that overexerts itself physically may experience heat stroke. Running alongside a bicycle for extended periods can be particularly dangerous. Being left alone in an overheated car can be just as hazardous.

A dog suffering from heat stroke pants heavily and is wobbly on its feet or is unable to get up at all. Its ears and nose are very hot and dry. The dog is unresponsive and extremely thirsty.

What to Do?
Immediately move the dog to a shady spot or a cool room. Apply wet, cold compresses for additional relief. Offer water, but not ice-cold water. If the dog does not show signs of improvement within five to ten minutes, transport it to a clinic or your veterinarian's office as quickly as possible.

● *Circulatory Collapse*
Several different problems can cause a circulatory collapse: overheating (See "Heat Stroke"), physical overexertion, a severe viral infection, an accident, or poisoning.

A dog suffering from a circulatory collapse lies on its side and doesn't react very much to any stimulation. The gums and the conjunctivas in the eyes are very pale, almost white. The dog's breathing is flat, and the rate of breathing increases.

What to Do?
If possible, place the dog on a flat surface with its head lower than its pelvis. Transport the dog as quickly as possible to a clinic or your veterinarian.

TIP

If a dog is unconscious, transport it on its side. You need another person to help you transport a large dog. (See previous page.)

95

Index